Step by Step
MRI

Step by Step MRI

J Jagan Mohan Reddy
MD DMRD
Professor and Head
Department of Radiology and Imageology
Nizam's Institute of Medical Sciences
(A University established under the State Act)
Hyderabad, Andhra Pradesh, 500082

V Prasad
BSc CRA PGDRIT
MRI Technologist
Department of Radiology and Imageology
Nizam's Institute of Medical Sciences
(A University established under the State Act)
Hyderabad, Andhra Pradesh, 500082

Taylor & Francis
Taylor & Francis Group
LONDON AND NEW YORK
A MARTIN DUNITZ BOOK

First published in India in 2005
Jaypee Brothers Medical Publishers (P) Ltd, New Delhi, India.
EMCA House, 23/23B Ansari Road, Daryaganj, New Delhi 110 002, India
Phones: 23272143, 23272703, 23282021, 232456727, Fax: +91-011-23276490
e-mail: jpmedpub@del2.vsnl.net.in, Visit our website: www.jaypeebrothers.com

First published by Martin Dunitz, a member of the Taylor & Francis Group plc in 2005. Exclusively distributed worldwide (excluding the Indian Subcontinent) by Martin Dunitz, a member of the Taylor & Francis Group plc.

Tel.: +44 (0) 1235 828600
Fax.: +44 (0) 1235 829000
E-mail: info@dunitz.co.uk
Website: http://www.dunitz.co.uk

A CIP record for this book is available from the British Library.

ISBN 1 84184 537X

Distributed in North and South America by

Taylor & Francis
2000 NW Corporate Blvd
Boca Raton, FL 33431, USA

Within Continental USA
Tel.: 800 272 7737; Fax.: 800 374 3401
Outside Continental USA
Tel.: 561 994 0555; Fax.: 561 361 6018
E-mail: orders@crcpress.com

Distributed in the rest of the world (excluding the Indian Subcontinent) by
Thomson Publishing Services
Cheriton House
North Way
Andover, Hampshire SP10 5BE, UK
Tel.: +44 (0)1264 332424
E-mail: salesorder.tandf@thomsonpublishingservices.co.uk

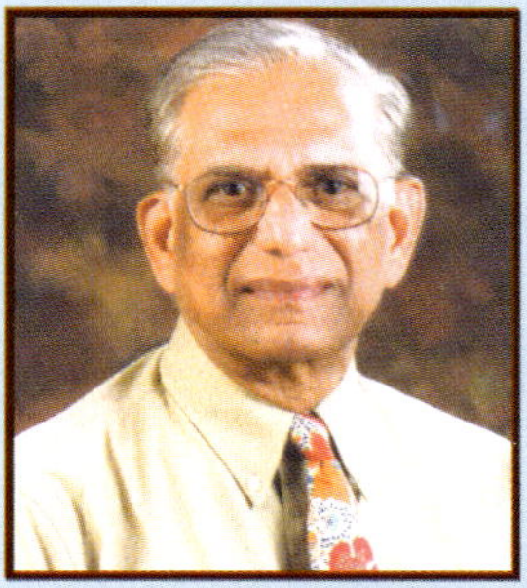

Dedicated to
Padmasri Prof Kakarla Subbarao
Director and Vice Chancellor, NIMS,
Hyderabad

Foreword

It is with great pride and gratification that I pen these few words as a "Foreword" to this master piece. Dedication, devotion, determination and a little detachment from the family activities are essential to produce such a creative work.

As I know the authors quite intimately for almost two decades, their impeccable loyalty and commitment to their chosen speciality are exemplary.

Since the first application of MRI in clinical practice in early 1980, phenominal developments have taken place. It has emerged as the best non-radiation imaging method of investigation. I know, quite a number of technologists, even Radiologists and other MRI specialists cannot really follow the basics, protocols, but operate and interpret the images.

This book really serves to present greater comprehension and to put in the authors own words "a clear-cut understanding of the principles underlying MRI for fruitful and effective use".

I am sure this book serves as a Bible to all those who are involved in imaging sciences and I do hope that the authors keep upgrading the latest developments in their next editions. May the scientific world derive benefit by going through this volume.

I do appreciate the sincerity, loyalty and generosity of the authors for dedicating this invaluable piece to me.

Prof Kakarla Subbarao
Director

Preface

From the initial observation that dense material attenuates X-rays, the complex field of medical imaging has developed. With the knowledge of relative densities of various tissues, radiologists and other physicians have used radiography to diagnose disease in every body part and organ system. Nearly two decades old clinical Magnetic Resonance Imaging offers diagnostic power far beyond that of radiographic density or any other principle of imaging. MRI utilizes several different principles alone or in combination to address a medical question. A clear-cut understanding of the principles underlying MRI is essential for its fruitful and effective use. The success of MRI in practice mainly lies in its clarity and logicality. It is becoming increasingly difficult to keep pace with the developments in MRI. MRI requires a multitude of operating parameter decisions and improper choices can result in impaired image quality leading to wrong diagnosis.

There are several books on MRI but they are all from foreign authors. Some Indian authors also published books on Radiology and Imageology, in which MRI is one chapter or a part of it. Realizing the important role of MRI in the field of Imageology without the effects of radiation, we have made an attempt in this book exclusively on MRI to give a comprehensive presentation of the various principles and techniques of MRI.

While preparing this book we have taken into account our experiences with the protocols which change from institution to institution, consultant to consultant, company to company and equipment to equipment, version to version and technologists to technologists, while however the basic fundamentals remain the same.

Chapter-1 is about Introduction

Chapter-2 deals with Basic Principles

Chapter-3 illustrates Components of MRI system

Chapter-4 relates to Contraindications and Patient Safety

Chapter-5 belongs to Pulse Sequences

Chapter-6 explains Tissue Characteristics

Chapter-7 handles Artifacts

The topics of Technical Factors Influencing the Image Quality, MRI Contrast Agents, Recent Advances in Pulse Sequences and Practical Imaging are dealt with in chapters 8, 9, 10 and 11

Suggestions, expert advice and constructive criticism are invited to enable us to handle them in our future editions.

J Jagan Mohan Reddy
V Prasad

Acknowledgements

For an employee whose services are needed round the clock that too in a premier institute like Nizam's Institute of Medical Sciences, which caters to patients from three southern states, writing a book is an uphill task and literally impossible. But our long cherished desire has become a reality with the kind encouragement, co-operation and guidance of our beloved Director, Prof K Subbarao. Our profound thanks go to our Director who always said 'OK' to all our ventures.

Any book particularly scientific in nature requires the assistance and co-operation from all the colleagues in the Department. Our sincere and heartfelt thanks are to the faculty, Residents and colleagues Mr Ch VVSN Murthy, Mr D Sanjeevaiah, who extended their unstinted support in preparing material for this book.

We express our sincere thanks to Mrs Sri Vani, Typist and Mr G Mohd Siraj Ahmed, PG Diploma in Radiography and Imaging Technology. We acknowledge, with thanks, the contribution of Mr K Damodar Naidu, Radiographer who wrote the Chapter on "Pulse sequences" and that of Mr Ibrahim Jamal Mohammed, a Radiographer based in United Kingdom.

We thank our family members and children who spared us with the requisite time to prepare this book.

Last but not least, our grateful thanks are to M/s SIEMENS, M/s Philips and M/s GE Wipro, whose MRI machines are the basis for this booklet.

Our special and sincere thanks are to M/s Jaypee Brothers Medical Publishers (P) Ltd., New Delhi, who have gracefully accepted to publish this booklet.

Contents

One

Introduction

The story of MRI is one of a long courtship between Physics and Medicine. In 1952, Dr Bloch from Stanford University and Dr Purcell from Harvard University were awarded the Nobel Prize for their work on what was then known as "Nuclear Magnetic Resonance (NMR)". However, the turning point came after 20 years with the advent of computers in medical imaging. By this time, the word 'nuclear' is substituted and it is now known as "Magnetic Resonance Imaging (MRI)".

The medical world had experienced a boom in 1973 when Lauterbur and Damadian, working independently, pronounced the potentiality of the science of Magnetic Resonance, in imaging the human body. Since then tremendous advances have taken place in the design and technology of magnetic resonance equipment, incorporating computer know-how and sophisticated electronics to provide sectional images of the human body with excellent delineation unparalleled in medical arena. This new diagnostic modality gives minute structural details of the human body utilizing the magnetic properties of the nuclei of atoms, mainly hydrogen in human tissues.

As a tribute to this endeavors, Dr Damadian received the National Medal of Technology from President Reagan in July

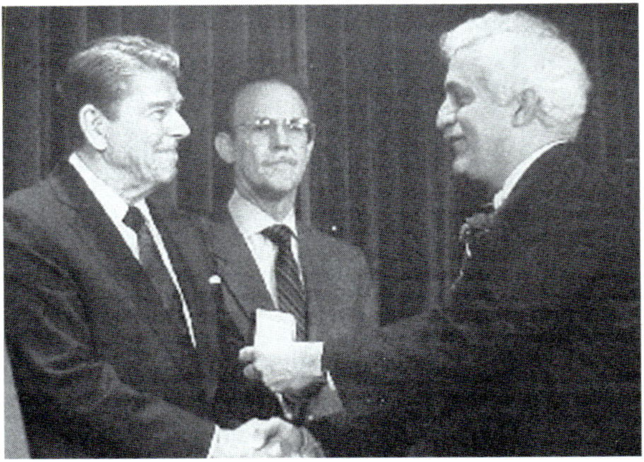

Fig. 1.1: Dr Damadian receives the National Medal of Technology from President Reagan in July15,1988; for his independent contributions in conceiving and developing the application of magnetic resonance technology to medical uses, including whole-body scanning and diagnostic imaging

15, 1988. The pioneers of the newly emerged imaging modality of the current era *viz.* Magnetic Resonance Imaging (MRI); an American Scientist, Lauterbur aged 74 years and a British scientist, Peter Mansfield aged 70 years are honoured with

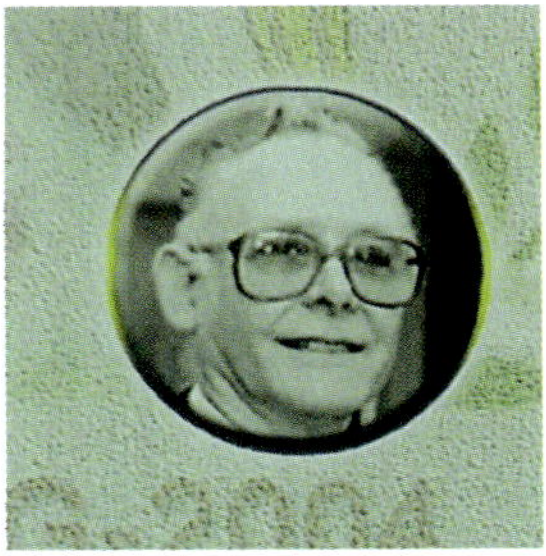

Fig. 1.2: Sir Peter Mansfield

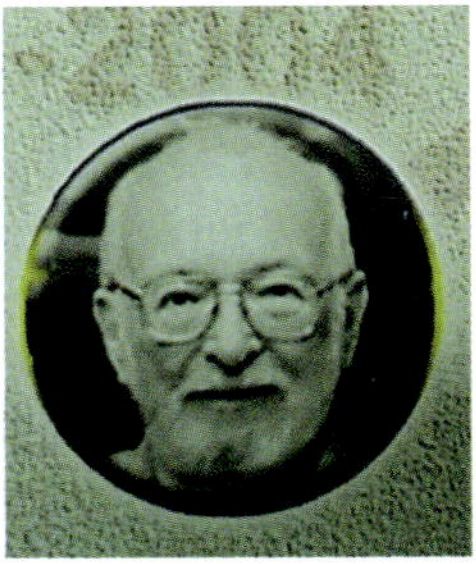

Fig. 1.3: Prof C Lauterbur

"Nobel Prize" on 10th December of the current year, i.e. 2003, for their outstanding contribution in the field of medicine (Diagnostic Radiology) which paved the way for the novel approach of the diagnosis of pathologies, disorders which are even obscured in various parts of the body and help the medical personnel in particular, in developing the corresponding suitable remedies in order to abate the sufferings of the mankind. Here we, on behalf of the mankind, are really indebted to the above personalities for their enviable innovation which proved to be quite helpful to a larger extent in mitigating the sufferings of the people.

Two

Basic Principles

THE BASICS

Electromagnetic Radiation (Fig. 2.1)

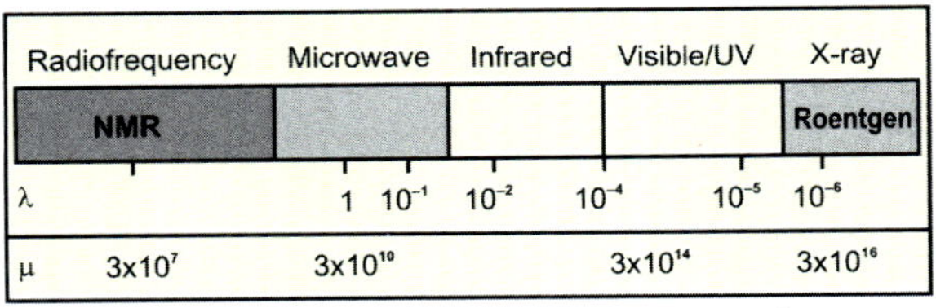

Fig. 2.1: Spectrum of electromagnetic radiation

As seen in Fig. 2.1 the radiofrequencies of the nuclear magnetic resonance (NMR) signals are 9 orders of magnitude smaller than the frequencies corresponding to the X-rays. Transmitted X-rays have been used for years to generate images of the human body. We will now show how NMR signals can be used to produce a very exciting new type of image. While X-ray images stem from interactions between the X-rays and the electron clouds of atoms, the NMR signals stem from the interaction of radiowaves with the atomic nuclei themselves.

Atoms consist of a nucleus surrounded by one or more electrons. The nucleus consists of one or more "positively charged protons" and also contains neutral particles called "neutrons".

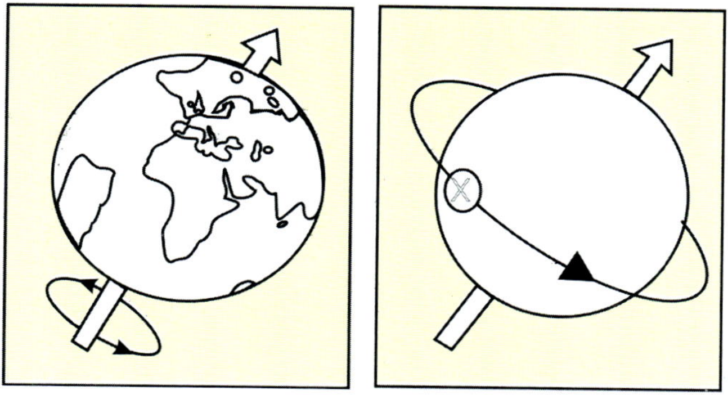

Fig. 2.2: Protons possess a positive charge; like the earth, they are constantly turning around on an axis and have their own magnetic field

Protons: The nucleus of the hydrogen atom has just one proton and no neutron. It has the highest sensitivity to magnetic resonance.

SPIN: Protons, neutrons, electrons and other particles possess a remarkable characteristic known as 'Spin'.

The spin of the atomic particles is depicted in Fig. 2.2.

MR Active Nuclei

Important MR active nuclei together with their atomic number and orientation are given in Fig. 2.3, some of which are used in MR spectroscopy.

Most abundantly available hydrogen nuclei is in the form of water given in Fig. 2.4.

Hydrogen Atom

Hydrogen atoms are abundantly present in the body.

The hydrogen nucleus is the MR active nucleus used in MRI. The hydrogen nucleus contains a single proton as shown in Fig. 2.5.

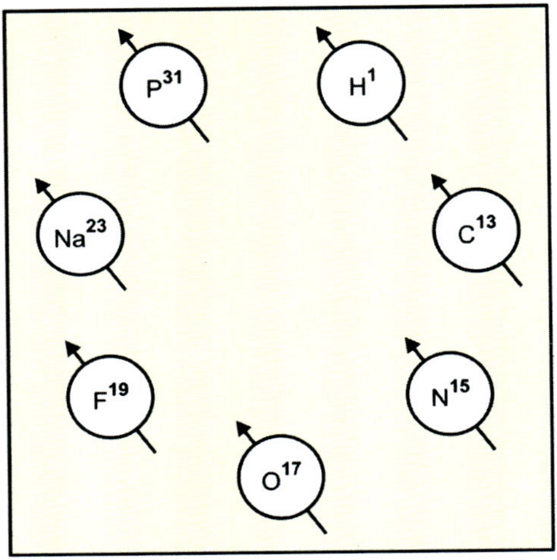

Fig. 2.3: Various MR active nuclei with their atomic number with linear alignment

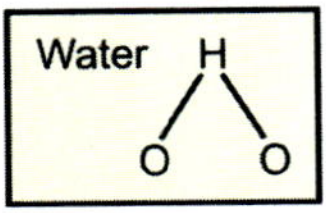

Fig. 2.4: The molecular structure of water (H_2O)

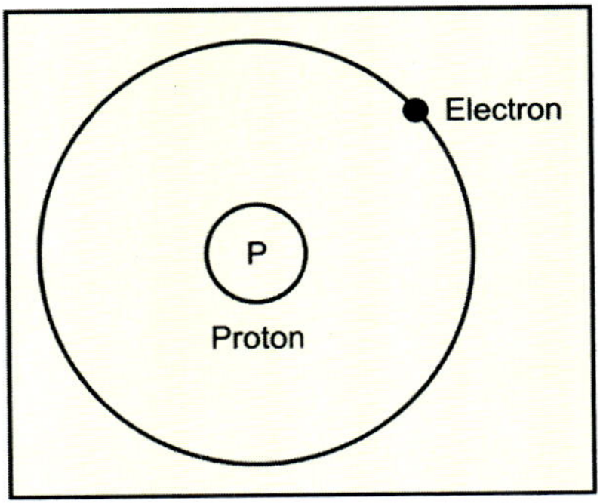

Fig. 2.5: Hydrogen atom

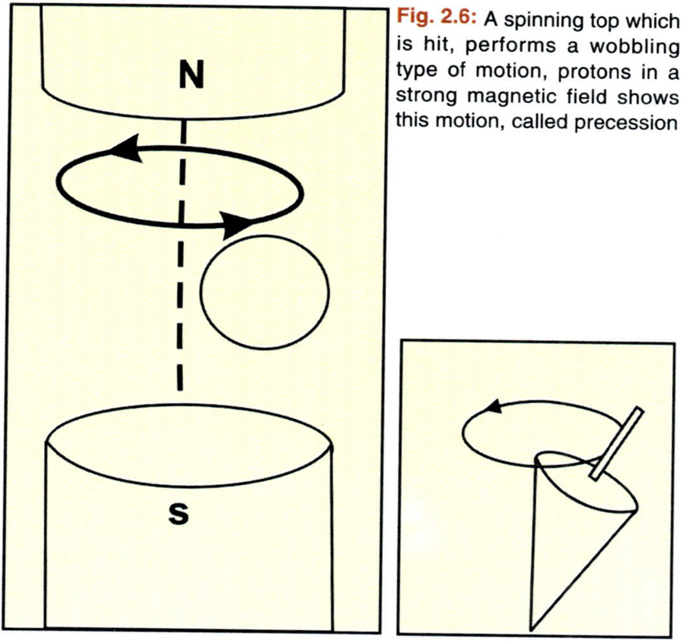

Fig. 2.6: A spinning top which is hit, performs a wobbling type of motion, protons in a strong magnetic field shows this motion, called precession

The nucleus of the hydrogen proton depicting its motion is shown in Fig. 2.6.

Positive charge, i.e. Proton—it spins at a very high speed.

This combination of spin and charge generates tiny magnetic field.

The strength and direction of this field is represented by a vector called 'magnetic moment'.

Vectors

A vector is a symbol representing the magnitude and direction of the magnetic field.

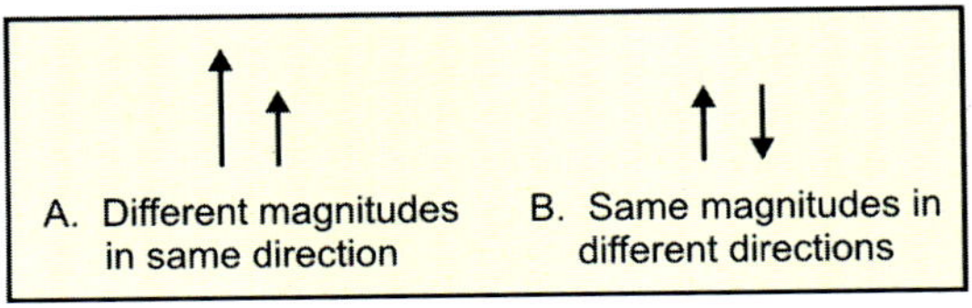

Fig. 2.7: Alignment of vectors with varying magnitudes

A vector is commonly represented by a directed line segment, i.e. an arrow which denotes its magnitude and its direction (Fig. 2.7).

(The orientation of the arrow is space corresponding to the direction of the vector quantity, the length of the arrow corresponding to the vector magnitude. Please remember that the arrow is merely a symbol for a real physical quantity).

Spin magnets behave like vectors. They exhibit a magnetic field that has both magnitude and direction.

Magnetic Moments

a. A rotating particle has an electric charge. Moving charges, as we know, are nothing more than electrical currents. An electric current has an associated magnetic field.
b. Where there is an electrical current, there is also a magnetic field.
c. Classically, the magnetic effect of a rotating charge or an electrical ring current is known as the magnetic moment.

It is like the earth constantly rotates around an axis and has its own magnetic field. Similarly, protons possessing a positive charge and continuous motion have their own magnetic field.

PRINCIPLE

The human body is a chemical composition of several elements, such as hydrogen, carbon, nitrogen, sodium, phosphorus, potassium, etc. in various chemical combinations. It has been observed that the atoms of some of these elements, have odd number of protons in their nuclei, possess magnetic properties. The magnetic properties of the protons of these elements have been utilized to produce magnetic resonance signals and images. The most abundant of these present in the human body are the protons of hydrogen atom in the form of water and various other organic compounds such as fats, fluids, cholesterol, etc.

What is MR?

When a patient is placed in the strong magnetic field in the MRI scanner, the hydrogen nucleus in the body, align with the applied external magnetic field when exposed to short burst of electromagnetic energy in the form of radiofrequency (RF) pulses (Fig. 2.8).

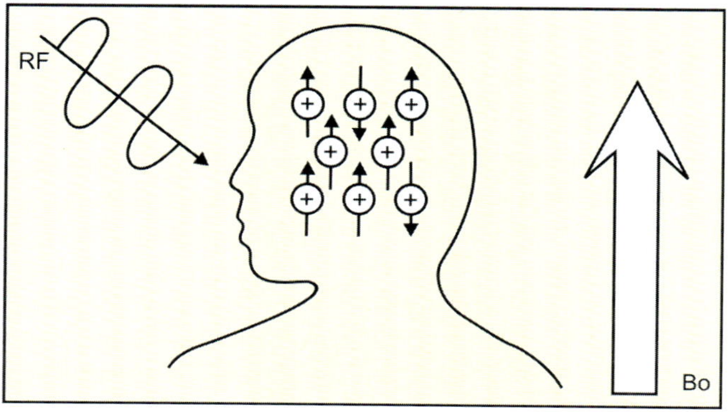

Fig. 2.8: Alignment of hydrogen nucleus in the human body when placed in strong magnetic field

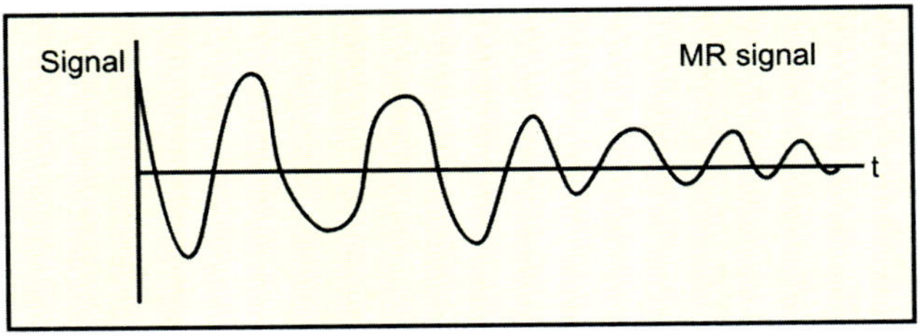

Fig. 2.9: Energy of the generated MR signal

The hydrogen nuclei in the patient's body absorb its energy and then generate MR signal. This process of absorbing energy is known as 'magnetic resonance'. It forms the basics of MR imaging (Fig. 2.9).

Magnetic Resonance

If radiofrequency equals the precessional frequency, then the phenomenon of resonance occurs.

Let us compare the resonance stimulations in MR with oscillations created by various tuning forks (Fig. 2.10). When the tuning fork is vibrated or perturbed, it begins to oscillate at a specific frequency relative to sound. The pitch corresponds to the oscillation frequency of the acoustic wave. When you introduce a second tuning fork having

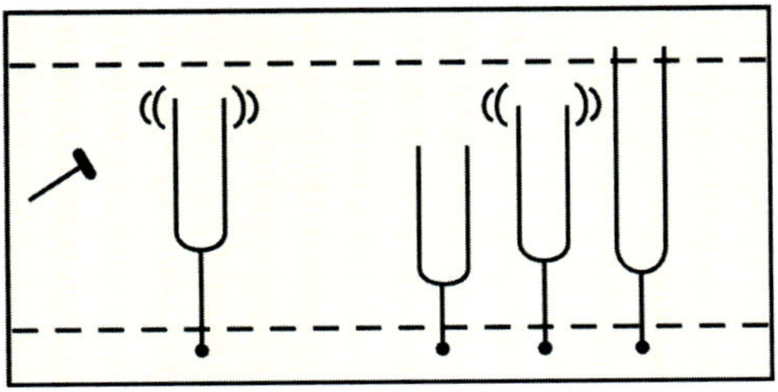

Fig. 2.10: Resonance stimulation with oscillation induced by tuning forks of various frequencies

the same frequency of the former, it starts oscillating in response to the acoustic waves emitted from the former tuning fork. At that moment, the tuning forks are said to be in "resonance".

Hydrogen nuclei (with single proton) in the absence of external interference, are in random motion and their magnetic moment cancel each other resulting in overall 'null or zero magnetization'.

According to the Law of Quantum mechanics, in the presence of an external magnetic field, the spinning nuclei may align themselves in two directions *viz.* parallel or antiparallel to the external magnetic field applied. Therefore, when the patient is placed inside the magnetic field, the hydrogen nuclei (protons) in the body get aligned in proper orientation and this leads to the patient being magnetized which in turn emits signals which are captured by the receiver and after a series of processing, transformation results in the formation of images on the screen (Fig. 2.11).

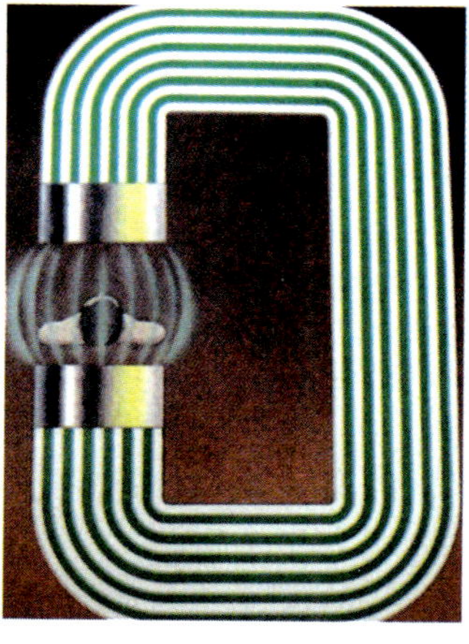

Fig. 2.11: The patient is placed in the center of the huge, powerful magnetic system

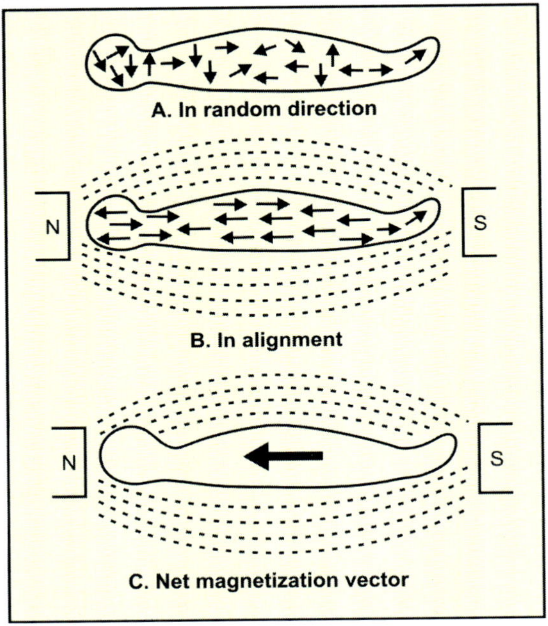

Fig. 2.12: Hydrogen protons in human body

These hydrogen protons in the human body are in a random orientation pointing in different directions as shown in Fig. 2.12A.

As shown in Fig. 2.12B under the influence of applied external magnetic field, the patient's tiny hydrogen proton magnets tend to align themselves in the direction of the external magnetic field.

Fig. 2.12C represents a bulk or net magnetization vector.

In conventional radiology or CT scan, the signal solitarily depends on one parameter, X-ray beam attenuation coefficient. In MRI, image is constructed with a set of signals. The image is generated by three factors.

The three parameters—Proton density.

T1, T2—Relaxation times.

The tiny magnets of the human body are then subjected to an impact of additional magnetic influences, in the form of radiofrequency (RF) waves, magnetic gradient coils, etc. to derive magnetic resonance signals. The MR signals obtained have a wide range of specificities, depending on the strength of the magnetic field, the frequency and duration of radiofrequency waves (pulse sequence), the magnetic gradients employed, the proton density, the element containing the protons, the chemical combination of elements, their molecular state, etc.

The various types of signals obtained are labeled as T1, T2 relaxation signals. The magnetic resonance signals have specific tissue characteristics. These are analyzed by a computer and reconstructed mathematically by a process known as "Fourier's transformation" into sectional images of the human body, accordingly, as T1 weighted image, proton density image, T2 weighted images.

The various types of images exhibit specific tissue characteristics, by which the tissues can be distinguished.

The behaviour of individual magnetic moments cannot be measured.

The signal measured in MRI is produced by the sum of all magnetic moments called "net magnetization".

Net magnetization points in the same direction as the scanned main magnetic field.

PRECESSION FREQUENCY

Every hydrogen nucleus which constitutes the net magnetization vector (NMV) spins on its own axis. The

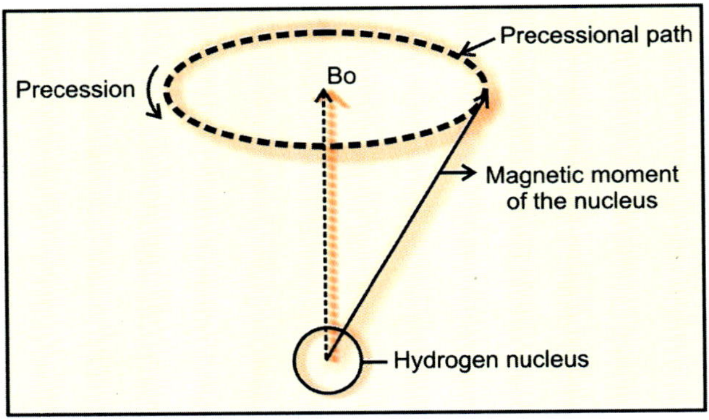

Fig. 2.13: Precession

influence of external magnetic field (Bo) produces an additional spin or wobble of NMV around Bo. Like a spinning top, proton shows wobbling type of motion called "precession". This secondary spin is known as 'precession' causes the magnetic moment to follow a circular path around the magnetizing field (Bo). This path is known as the "precessional path" and the speed with which the NMV wobbles around Bo is known as the "precessional frequency". The unit of precessional frequency is "Mega Hertz (MHz).

The precision frequency can be calculated by the Larmor's equation, and is higher in stronger magnetic fields.

Larmor's Equation (Table 2.1)

ω	=	γ	* Bo
Precessional frequency		Hydrogen (42.6) MH_2T	Magnetic field strength

ω (omega)	=	The precessional frequency in MHz
γ (gamma)	=	The gyromagnetic ratio of hydrogen at 1T is 42.58 MHz
Bo	=	The magnetic field strength of magnet (in Tesla).

Table 2.1: Gyromagnetic ratio (γ) of various nuclei

Nucleus	*Gyromagnetic ratio MHz/T*
H^1	42.58
C^{13}	10.71
P^{31}	17.12

Table 2.2: The Larmor's frequency at various field strengths

Field strength	*Frequency*
0.5T	22.28 MHz
1.0T	42.58 MHz
1.5T	63.9 MHz

The precessional frequency is often called the "Larmor's frequency" (Table 2.2). It is directly proportional to the strength of the magnetic field.

Radiofrequency or Excitation

If radiofrequency pulse having the same frequency as that of the precessing nuclei is applied, the precessing path of the nuclei will be at right angles and thus it spirals away which resembles like the wobbling of a spinning top.

Hence, radiofrequency pulse at Larmor's frequency has the following effects:

1. The RF pulse provides sufficient energy to some of the hydrogen nuclei to align antiparallel to main magnetic field, they in turn cancel out the magnetic effect of remaining parallel nuclei and thus decrease the amount of longitudinal magnetization. The decrease in longitudinal magnetization depends upon the strength and duration of RF pulse.
2. With the decrease of longitudinal magnetization, there is a corresponding gradual increase in magnetization in transverse plane (B1). This is because the protons which were in 'out of phase' are now precessing 'in phase'.

   Resonance occurs at 42 MHz when Bo = 1T

Loud Noise during MR Procedure

The continuous movement of the gradient coils during the examination is very loud. Patients could use ear plugs during MR examination to make it tolerable.

In the Magnetic Field

Each magnetic field exerts a force on magnetic and magnetizable particles, including the spin magnets. The effect of this force is depicted by magnetic field lines (a).

The strength of this force at each location in space is known as "magnetic induction". However, in MR Technology, the term "magnetic field strength" is commonly used. The field strength is expressed in units of Tesla; (T:SI unit) or Gauss (G:T = 10,000 G).

Tesla is approximately 20,000 times stronger than the earth's magnetic field.

A magnetic field of uniform field strength is known as a "homogenous magnetic field" (Fig. 2.14).

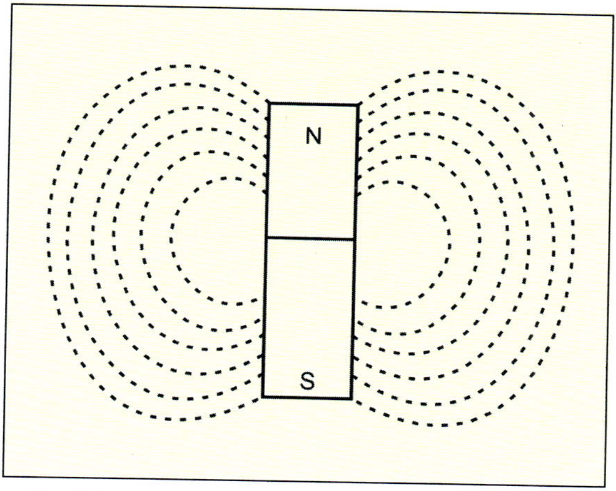

Fig. 2.14: Field lines in homogenous magnetic field

The field lines of homogenous field are drawn at distance, straight lines running in parallel (b).

When the magnetic field does not vary with time, it is known as "static field".

Three

Components of MRI System

INTRODUCTION

Open MRI units have two advantages that they can be used for claustrophobic patients, and they provide imaging guidance for interventional procedures.

Open units image the patient in larger-bore or c-shaped magnets rather than the closed narrow tunnel used in conventional units. These magnets are weaker (0.1-0.3 T) than the closed units and their basic contrast results in some limitation in anatomic and spatial resolution (Figs 3.1 and 3.2).

What is meant by high and low field strength MRI?

Manufactures produce magnets of varying strengths. The most common magnetic field strengths clinically are 0.3, 0.5, 1.0, 1.5 and 3 Tesla. Magnets of 1.0 Tesla or higher are treated high-field strength which generate higher signals and usually more appealing images than lower-field strength units.

Therefore, the high-field strength units generally offer more esthetic and diagnostic images than the open units and should preferably be used whenever possible.

It is easy to answer to the question about the ideal horse-power for a motor bike.

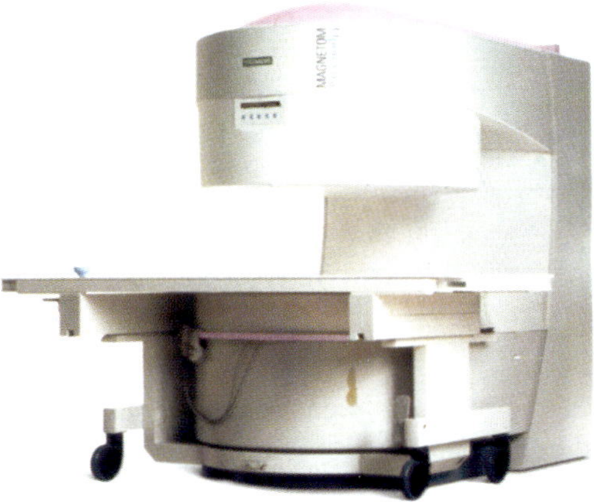

Fig. 3.1: Open MRI unit (Courtesy of Siemens)

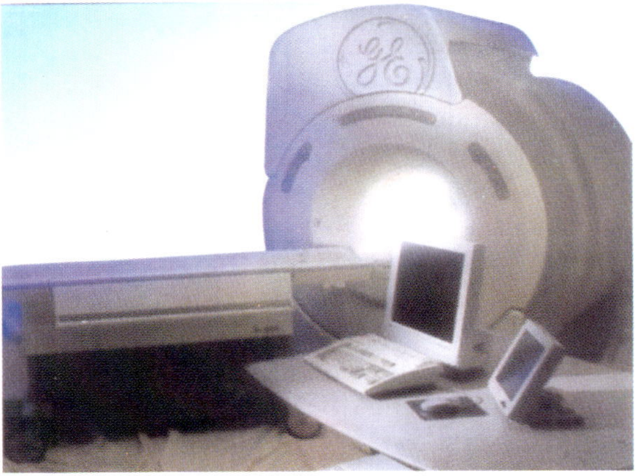

Fig. 3.2: A modern MRI unit (Courtesy of GE Medical Systems)

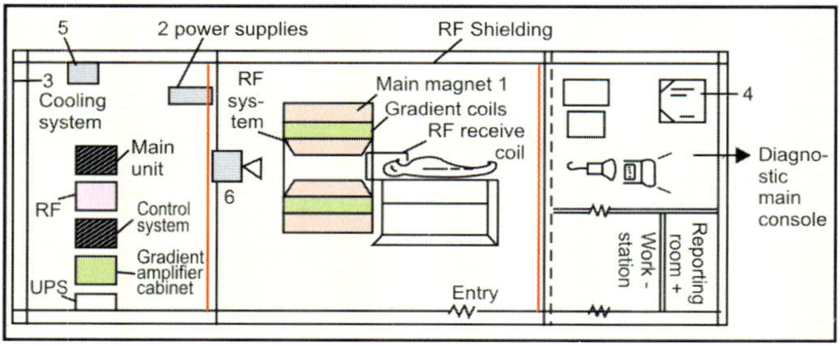

Fig. 3.3: System of a superconductive MRI system

High-field strength systems have a better spatial resolution and are used for spectroscopy.

The Components of the MRI System (Fig. 3.3)

1. The magnet which is a key element of the MRI system. It is integrated into the system which also includes; (i) the RF and (ii) Gradient system.
2. Power supplies
3. A computer system
4. A documentation system
5. Cooling system
6. Monitoring camera

Camera can be placed to monitor a patient inside the magnet bore.

Magnet room has to be shielded with a Faraday's cage to prevent interferences between outside frequency waves and those used with MR equipment.

Documentation

According to the tasks involved, computed data and reconstructed images are stored either in:

- a fixed storage medium—Magnetic Hard Disks
- a removable storage medium—Magneto Optical Disks.

Camera

The MR Images are exposed on X-ray film with the laser camera connected to the MRI system.

Magnet

The main component of MRI is, of course, the magnet, available in three types—*viz.*, the permanent magnets, electromagnets and superconducting magnets. The homogeneous magnetic field required for MR Imaging is generated by a strong magnet. This magnet is the most important and expensive component of the MRI system.

a. *Permanent magnets:* Though simple and cheap to run, they are still extremely heavy and do not generate high fields (Fig. 3.4A).

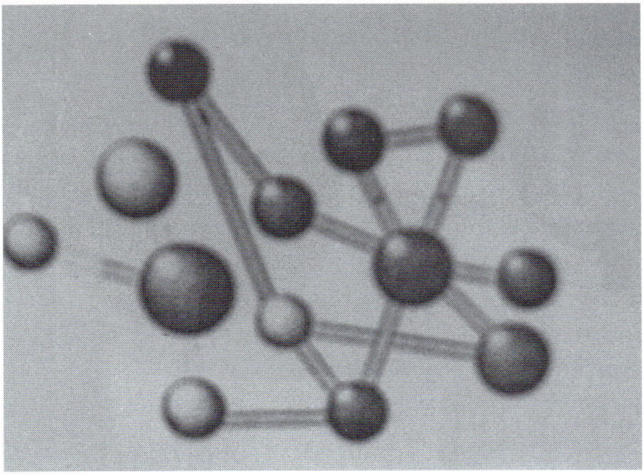

Fig. 3.4A: Molecular structure of permanent magnet

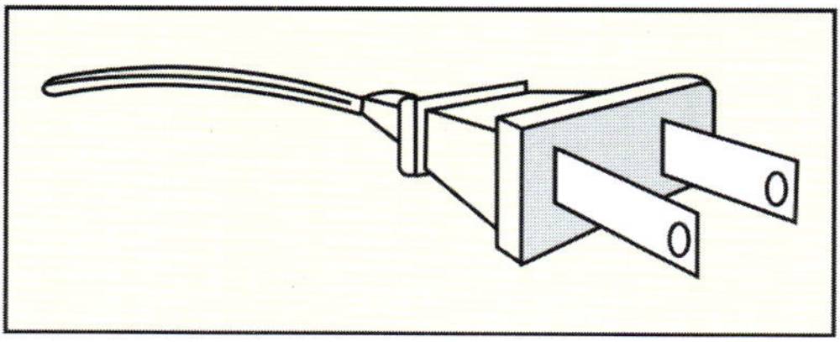

Fig. 3.4B: Resistive magnet

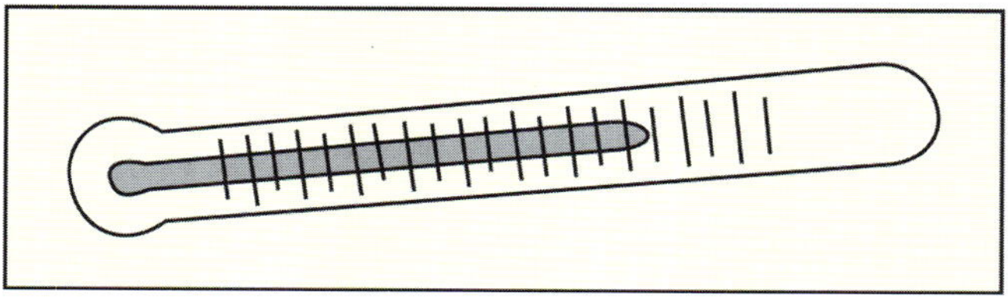

Fig. 3.4C: Superconductive magnet

b. *Resistive systems:* These are electromagnets wherein the magnetic field is generated by an electric current flowing through a coil (Fig. 3.4B). They have two major drawbacks. High electric and water consumption (cooling) and generate fields that are difficult to raise above 1.5 T.

c. *Superconductive magnets* (Fig. 3.4C): These are also electromagnets, made of materials with no electric resistance when placed at a temperature close to absolute zero (–273°C). They consume no power and allow stable and very high fields to be generated.

Their major drawback is running costs of cryogens (helium and nitrogen). However, they are more and more commonly used.

Coil

When the protons return to equilibrium, the signal is picked up by the receiver coil. The spins are stimulated by pulsed magnetic RF fields. These RF pulses are transmitted. The resulting RF signal has to be received since it contains the information necessary for image reconstruction.

The types of coils described below are the most commonly used (Figs 3.5A to C).

- Volume coils: Head/body coil
- Surface/local coils: (orbits, ear, wrist, shoulder, joints, etc).
- Phased array coils (CTL, TORSO array, etc).
- Body coil is fixed inside the magnet (examination of thorax, abdomen+pelvis, thigh, leg, body Angio).

Surface coils can be placed closed to region of interest (circular, rectangular, extremity, wraparound) which gives high signal to noise ratio (SNR) since being close to the anatomy.

The correct choice of a coil gives the best signal to noise ratio (SNR) in the region of interest.

- Volume coils both transmit and receive radiofrequency (RF) pulses and are specially called 'Transceivers'.
- Surface and local coils are traditionally used to improve the signal to noise ratio (SNR) when imaging the structure near to the skin surface. They only receive only signal.
- *Phased array coils*: It consists of multiple coils and receivers. It is used for larger areas.

SHIELDING

- Magnetic shielding is required to protect the surrounding environment from the effects of fringe fields which surround a magnet.

To maintain magnetic field homogeneity, shielding is necessary for the field to be protected from being distorted by the external environment.

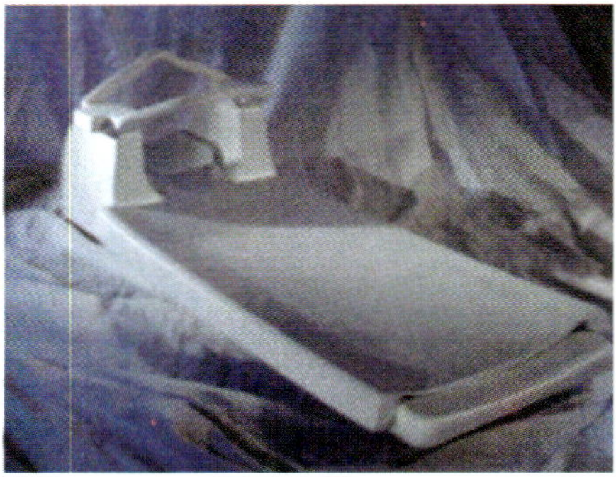

Fig. 3.5A: Quadrature CTL phased array coil

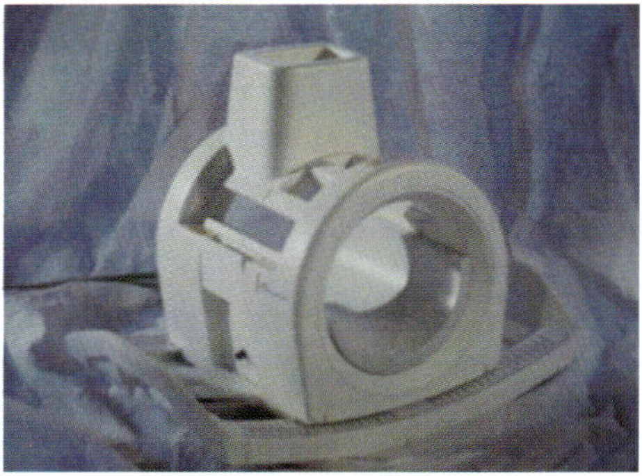

Fig. 3.5B: Extremity coil

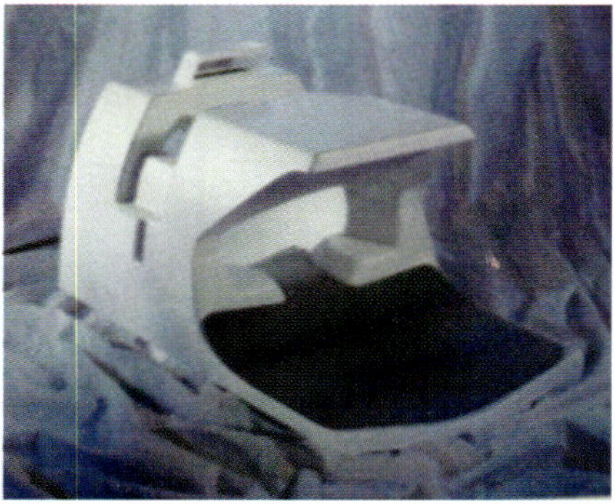

Fig. 3.5C: NV array coil

RF Shielding

The MRI signal is relatively weak. Hence, small external RF interferences can significantly degrade the image quality. As a result, MRI systems generally require that the imaging room be shielded from external sources of RF energy. For most of the systems, this involves building RF shielding into the side walls, floor and ceiling of the MR site. RF shielding also prevents the RF signal generated during MR measurements from being disturbed by radio signals outside the MR room.

1. Shimming
2. Gradient.

Shimming

Better homogeneity can be achieved by electrical and mechanical adjustments by a process known as "shimming".

Correction of inhomogeneity of the magnetic field produced by the main magnet of MRI system is necessary due to imperfections in the magnet or due to the presence of external ferromagnetic objects.

The important quality for a magnet is "homogeneity" of its main magnetic field. Inhomogeneities distort the spatial encoding which in turn adversely affects the slice geometry. The MR image will show distortions in the slice plane.

In order to prevent this type of image errors, the magnet system has to be adjusted during system installation to local conditions or deviations in unit spread prevailing in the unit. A process called shimming is used. We differentiate between Active and Passive shimming.

Active Shimming

Several shim coils are attached to a shim tube. Small static currents with different amplitudes and polarity are adjusted for the shim. The small magnetic fields which are generated compensate for small inhomogeneities of the main field. After the shim, the main field of a superconducting magnet will vary by a few ppm (parts per million) only within a measuring field having a diameter of 50 cm approximately.

Passive Shimming

Small iron plates are attached to the magnet. Their strategic placement compensates for inhomogeneities or distortions in the magnetic field. This may involve changing the configuration of the magnet or the addition of shim coils (active shimming) or small pieces of steel (passive shimming).

Gradients

Special coils called *gradient coils* vary the strength of the magnetic field, frequency and phase of the electromagnetic wave in the transverse (X and Y axes) and longitudinal (Z axis) planes.

Gating

Cardiac Triggering

In cardiac imaging, the acquisition is generally triggered by an electrocardiogram and is tied to the RR interval. This effectively eliminates the blurring and artifact problem inherent in cardiac imaging, although it limits imaging strategies (ECG, Pg (peripheral gating)).

Cardiac gating uses the programmed TR to deliver the RF pulse and then monitors the cardiac cycle to determine which signal it uses for reconstruction.

Cardiac gating uses the electrical signal detected by leads placed on patient's chest to trigger each RF excitation pulse.

Respiratory Gating

It is used to suppress breathing motion.

Acquisition takes place only during the "gate" when the respiratory movements are minimal. It is relatively effective at minimizing the effects of thoracic motion, but results in substantial increase in imaging time and hence, is not commonly employed.

Respiratory Triggering

In analogy to cardiac triggering, respiratory triggering can also be used to generate an electric signal upon expiration to start data acquisition.

Peripheral Gating (Pegating)

Pegating uses a photo sensor attached to either finger or toe.

Gating and respiratory compensation are commonly used to examine the chest and abdomen, and also used in imaging of brain (CSF flow, spinal cord and in cine).

Breath Holding and Abdominal Compression

Both techniques are employed whenever short acquisition sequences are employed, thereby minimizing the strain of the patient (Figs 3.6 and 3.7).

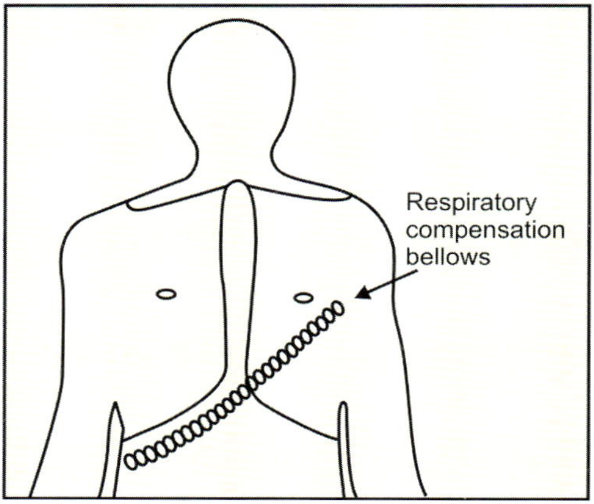

Fig. 3.6: Placement of the bellows

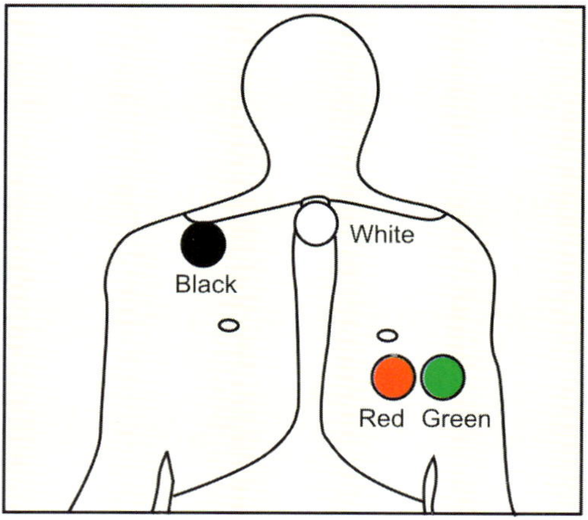

Fig. 3.7: Placement of the gating leads

MR COMPATIBLE CONTRAST MEDIA INJECTOR (MED RAD)

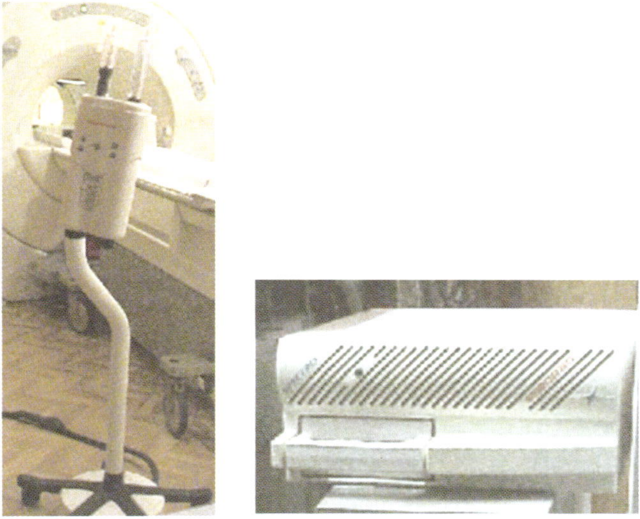

Fig. 3.8: MR compatible contrast media injector (Med Rad)

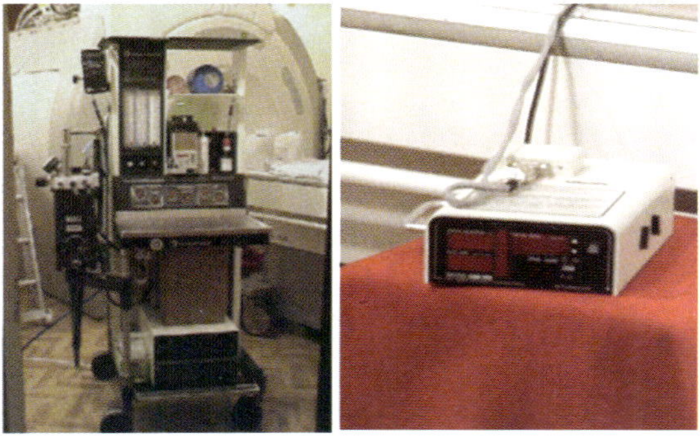

Pulse oximeter

Fig. 3.9: MR compatible anaesthesia equipment (Boyle's apparatus—Excel 210)

Quality Control (QC)

Quality control comprises the qualitative or quantitative measurements or tests of performance of an instrument or

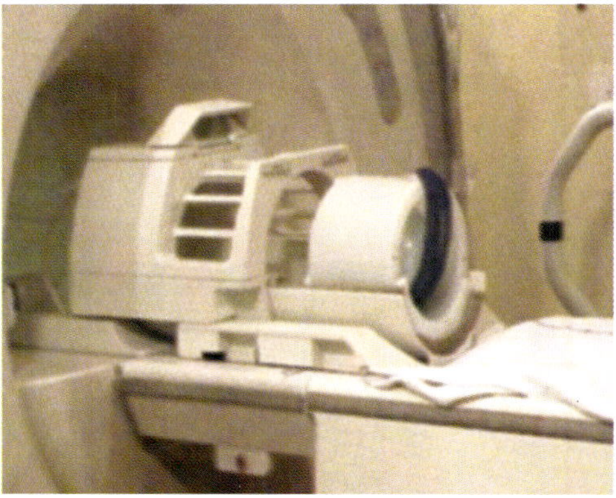

Fig. 3.10A: Phantom placed in the head coil

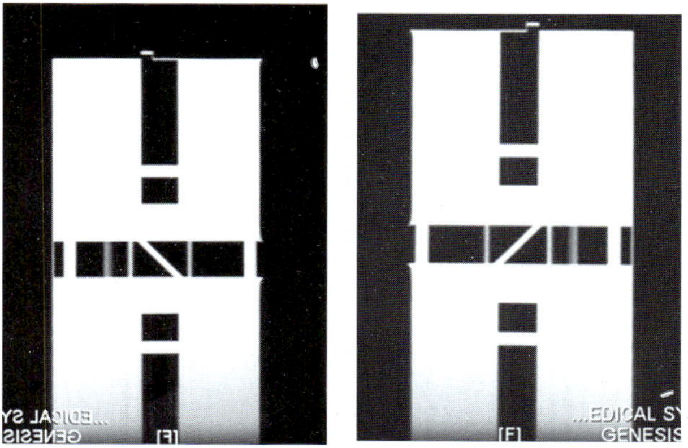

Fig. 3.10B: Image of DQA (daily quality assurance) Phantom coronal view

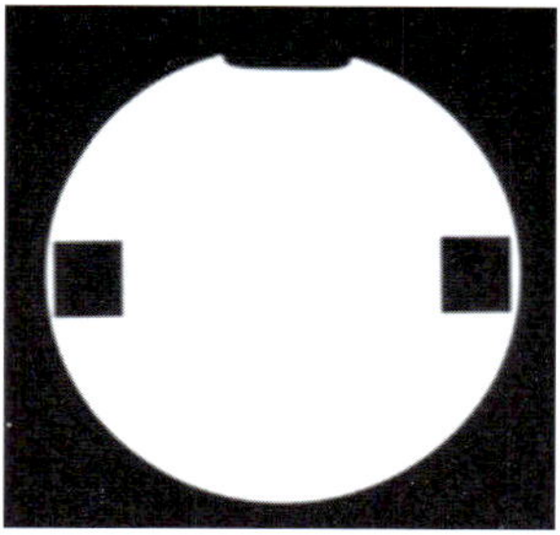

Fig. 3.10C: Image of DQA (daily quality assurance) Phantom axial view

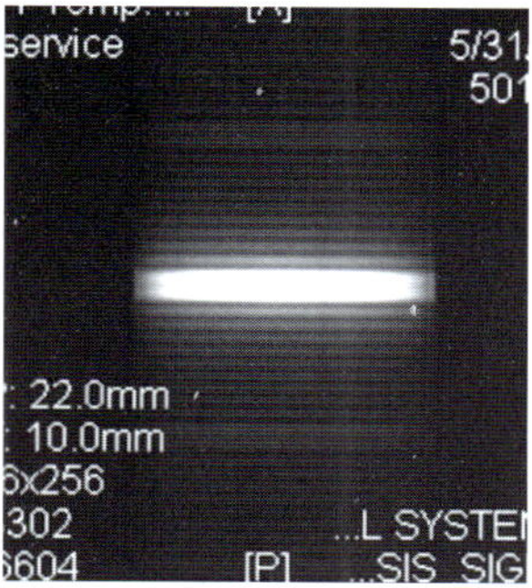

Fig. 3.10D: System performance test (SPT) scan image for head

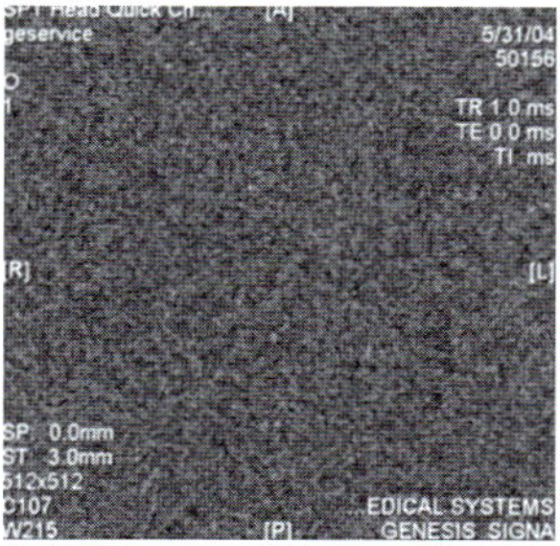

Fig. 3.10E: Noise scan

program and the determination of adequacy and acceptability of performance. This includes the set of operation (programming, coordinating) intend to maintain or to improve quality (ISO definition). In other words, as applied to diagnostic procedures, it covers monitoring, of all characteristics of performance that can be defined, measured and controlled.

Quality Assurance (QA)

The application of a service of quality control steps at multiple stages of a procedure to verify that all aspects of the procedure are of acceptable quality. The ISO definition is—all those planned and systematic actions necessary to provide adequate confidence that a structure, system or component will perform satisfactory in service.

Many of these tasks can be carried out by MR technologist. More extensive quality assurance should be performed periodically by qualified service engineer.

Quality Assurance in MRI

In order to get optimum image quality from a MRI system, a set of tests at regular interval alongwith the preventive maintenance measures are mandatory. The report of acceptance testing of the system (e.g. physical inventory, radiofrequency shielding verification, cryogenic fluid consumption, magnetic field in homogeneity, signal to noise ratio (SNR) or different coils, gradient coils, gradient strength linearity, provisions of image acquisition and image processing software, acoustic noise measurements and functioning of hard copy camera should be taken into account. All QA measures should be directed to get better image quality parameters.

The daily test ensures the smooth functioning of the system avoiding inconvenience to the patient. Daily tests take only 20 minutes and are carried out by the technologist every morning before the patient examination is resumed.

Four

Contraindications and Patient Safety

MR EXAMINATION PROCEDURE

Identity

Prior to any examination being performed, the identity of the patient must be checked by the technologist.

Patients arriving into MRI Department are often worried or apprehensive and this may make it difficult for them to understand the instructions or may produce an apparently aggressive attitude. In such cases, the technologist should convince amicably and soft tone of voice often do a great deal of comfort and gives the patient confidence that he/she is in an efficient hand.

The technologist should make every effort to obtain the willing cooperation of the patient consent. Children and uncooperative patients should be sedated before examination.

- Before entering the equipment room, the patient must wear a hospital gown and should remove all personal possessions such as watch, wallet, keys, hair pins, jewels, coils, removable dental bridge work, etc. Even credit cards and cell phones must be secured as the scanner will erase the information on them.
- Wheelchair and trolleys (MR noncompatible) must always be kept outside the magnet room.

The patient is made to lie down on a table. This table then passes through a tunnel within the equipment. Inside the tunnel, it is quite noisy when the scanning is going on. The region of interest is positioned at the center of the magnet. The patient can hear the voice of the radiologist or technologist and can respond. While the patient lies within the tunnel, images of the interested regions are taken from different angles. These images can be seen on a computer screen. The entire procedure takes 30 to 45 minutes approximately depending upon the strength of the magnetic field and the parameters set on.

It is most important that the patient should remain relaxed and completely still during the scan. The patient can resume the routine activities after getting the scan done.

- The patient should always be informed as to what is going to happen and what he/she is expected to do, so that he/she can cooperate as much as possible.
- The patient should not wear makeup because some products may contain metallic particles.
- The patient should be covered with a lightweight blanket.
- The patient must be made comfortable as far as possible because if the patient is in pain or in distress, it is unlikely that he will be able to remain still for long.
- *Explanation*: A detailed explanation of the exam to be performed (to be informed to the patient) to give the patient, particularly as to how long the procedure will take.
- The technologist from the start of examination/procedure should make an effort to remember the name of the patient with whom he or she is dealing and use it.
- Clear instructions regarding breathing or swallowing should be given and rehearsed to ensure that the patient does hold his breath or swallow when required to do so.

Due to the high magnetic field strengths used during MRI examination, certain patients are unsuitable for imaging. These include patients who have:

- Aneurysm clips (Older Ferromagnetic types)
- Cardiac pacemakers
- Patients with otologic implants and ocular implants
- Cochlear implants
- Metallic foreign bodies, especially within the eye.

Patient Screening

The following items can interfere with MR imaging and some can be hazardous to your safety. Please check if you have any of the following MR incompatible objects:

- Cardiac pacemaker/pacemaker lead wires
- Brain aneurysm clips
- Aortic clips
- Implanted neurostimulators or lead wires
- Artificial heart valve
- Insulin pump
- Electrodes
- Hearing aids
- IUD (Intrauterine Device)
- Shunts
- Joint replacements
- Fractured bones treated with metal rods, metal plates, pins, screws, nails or clips
- Harrington rod
- Bone or joint pins
- Prosthesis
- Metamesh
- Wire sutures

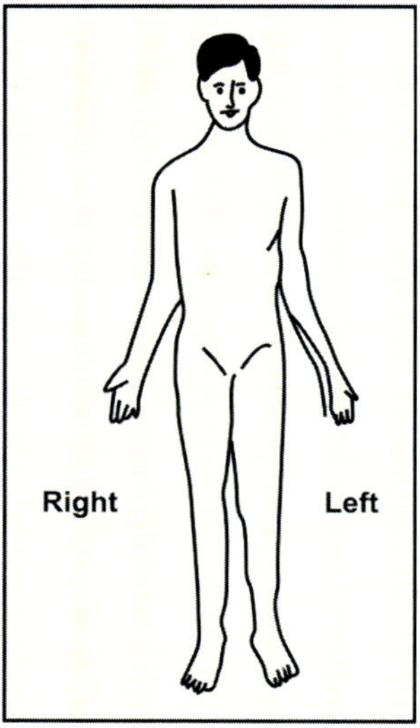

Fig. 4.1: To mark the location of any metal inside the body

- Sharpnel
- Dentures
- Metal silvers in the eyes
- Cochlear implants
- Tattoo eyeliner
- Others

On the drawing in Fig. 4.1, please mark the location of any metal "inside" the body.

Screening Prior to Scanning

- Glasses
- Removable dental work
- Hearing aid
- Jewellery

- Watch
- Wallet or money clip
- Pens or pencils
- Keys
- Coins
- Pocket knife
- Metal zippers or buttons
- Belt buckle
- Shoes
- Magnetic strip cards
- Credit cards, bank cards
- Hair pins or barrettes
- Metal bra hooks
- Bra and girdle underwear support
- Sanitary belt
- Safety pins

Patient Positioning

Positioning of the patient can affect the safety of the scan procedure.

Improper positioning can result in sunburn—like burns.

Precautions to be Undertaken

In order to maintain a safer scan environment, the following precautions are to be taken:

- MRI systems are equipped with laser alignment lights.
- Exposing eyes to the laser alignment lights may result in eye injury.
- Do not stare directly into the laser beam.
- Instruct the patients to close their eyes during land marking in order to avoid eye exposure to the alignment light while the laser light is "ON".

- Do not leave the laser beam ON after you position the patient.
- Place foams between the patient and the bore wherever a portion of the body comes in contact with the bore.
- Ensure that the patient does not touch the magnet bore.
- Orient the patient (head first or feet first) to minimize the length of the cable in the bore.
- For larger patients, use wide patient straps to secure the arms, preventing them from touching the bore.

EFFECTS OF RF POWER

The RF pulses used in MR causes tissues to absorb RF power under certain conditions. This may cause tissue heating. The amount of heating depends on several factors such as patient size and pulse-sequence timing.

Before the patient is being scanned, the computer estimates the level of heating and compares it to the predetermined exposure limits. If the scan exceeds these limits, the system then adjusts the scan parameters before starting the scan. The complete estimate is based partially on patient weight. Therefore, take care to enter the patient's weight correctly to prevent excessive RF.

HAZARDS

Claustrophobia despite the fact that the patient lies in a confined space is rarely a serious problem.

MRI has not been proved to have any adverse effects on fetuses. However, some teams avoid using during the first trimester of pregnancy.

Till date, no harmful effects have been observed from magnetic influences.

QUENCHING

A magnet quench will result in several days of down time. So, do not press or push the button except in a real emergency. Do not test that button. It should be tested only by qualified service personnel. Quench button is located near the magnet.

Magnet Quench Hazards

Magnetic quench is indicated by a loud noise, warning message, dense white vapor (with vent failure), helium meter dropping considerably or the tilting of an image on the image screen.

- If the patient needs medical attention, press an emergency stop button on the console or magnet and remove the patient from the scan room.
- Evacuate the patient and personnel from the scan room and close the scan room door.

APPENDIX

Metallic Implants and Other Objects Tested for Deflection Forces: A Compilation of the Literature

Metallic Implant or Object	Deflection	Highest Field Strength	Reference
Aneurysm and Hemostatic Clips			
Drake (DR14, DR24) (Edward Weck and Co., Triangle Park, NJ)	Yes	1.44 T	9
Drake (DR16) (Edward Weck and Co., Triangle Park, NJ)	Yes	0.147 T	9
Drake (301 SS) (Edward Weck and Co., Triangle Park, NJ)	Yes	1.5 T	11
Downs multipositional (17-7 PH)	Yes	1.44 T	9
Gastrointestinal anastomosis clip			
Autosuture SGLA, (SS) (United States Surgical Corp., Norwalk, CT)	No	1.5 T	11
Heifetz (17-7 PH) (Edward Weck and Co., Triangle Park, NJ)	Yes	1.89 T	4
Heifetz (Elgiloy) (Edward Weck and Co., Triangle Park, NJ)	No	1.89 T	4
Hemoclip #10, (316L SS) (Edward Weck and Co., Triangle Park, NJ)	No	1.5 T	11
Hemoclip (Tantalum) (Edward Weck and Co., Triangle Park, NJ)	No	1.5 T	11
Housepian	Yes	0.147 T	9
Kapp (405 SS) (V. Mueller)	Yes	1.89 T	4

Contd...

Contd...

Metallic Implant or Object	*Deflection*	*Highest Field Strength*	*Reference*
Kapp curved (404 SS) (V. Mueller)	Yes	1.44 T	9
Kapp straight (404 SS) (V. Mueller)	Yes	1.44 T	9
Ligaclip #6, (316L SS) (Ethicon Inc., Sommerville, NJ)	No	1.5 T	11
Ligaclip (Tantalum) (Ethicon Inc., Sommerville, NJ)	No	1.5 T	11
Mayfield (301 SS) (Codman, Randolph, MA)	Yes	1.5 T	11
Mayfield (304 SS) (Codman, Randolph, MA)	Yes	1.89 T	4
McFadden (301 SS) (Codman, Randolph, MA)	Yes	1.5 T	11
Olivercrona	No	1.44 T	9
Pivot (17-7 PH) (V. Mueller)	Yes	1.89 T	4
Scoville (EN58J) (Downs Surgical Inc., Decatur, GA)	Yes	1.89 T	4
Stevens (50-4190, Silver alloy)	No	0.15 T	2
Sugita (Elgiloy) (Downs Surgical Inc., Decatur, GA)	No	1.89 T	4
Sundt-Kees (301 SS) (Downs Surgical Inc., Decatur, GA)	Yes	1.5 T	11
Sundt-Kees Multi-Angle (17-7 PH) (Downs Surgical Inc., Decatur, GA)	Yes	1.89 T	4
Surgiclip, Autosuture M-9.5 (SS) (United States Surgical Corp., Norwalk, CT)	No	1.5 T	11
Vari-Angle (17-7 PH) (Codman, Randolph, MA)	Yes	1.89 T	4
Vari-Angle McFadden (MP35N) (Codman, Randolph, MA)	No	1.89 T	4
Vari-Angle Micro (17-7PM SS) (Codman, Randolph, MA)	Yes	0.15 T	2

Contd...

Contd...

Metallic Implant or Object	*Deflection*	*Highest Field Strength*	*Reference*
Vari-Angle Spring (17-7PM SS) (Codman, Randolph, MA)	Yes	0.15 T	2
Yasargil (316 SS) (Aesculap)	No	1.89 T	4
Yasargil (Phynox) (Aesculap)	No	1.89 T	4
Dental Materials			
Brace Band (SS) (American Dental, Missoula, Montana)	No	1.5 T	11
Brace Wire (Chrome alloy) (Ormco Corp., San Marcos, CA)	Yes*	1.5 T	11
Dental amalgam	No	1.44 T	9
Silver points (Union Broach Co., Inc., New York, NY)	No	1.5 T	11
Permanent crown (Amalgam) (Ormco Corp., San Marcos, CA)	No	1.5 T	11
Intravascular Coils, Filters and Stents			
Amplatz IVC filter (Cook, Bloomington, IN)	No	4.7 T	13
Cragg nitinol spiral filter	No	4.7 T	13
Gianturco embolization coil (Cook, Bloomington, IN)	Yes	1.5 T	13
Gianturco bird nest IVC filter (Cook, Bloomington, IN)	Yes	1.5 T	13
Gianturco zig-zag stent (Cook, Bloomington, IN)	Yes	1.5 T	13
Greenfield vena cava filter, Stainless steel (Meditech, Watertown, MA)	Yes*	1.5 T	13
Greenfield vena cava filter, Titanium alloy (Ormco, Glendora, CA)	No	1.5 T	13
Gunther IVC filter (William Cook, Europe)	Yes	1.5 T	13

Contd...

Contd...

Metallic Implant or Object	*Deflection*	*Highest Field Strength*	*Reference*
Mass helical IVC filter (Medinvent, Lausanne, Switzerland)	No	4.7 T	13
Mass helical endovascular stent (Medinvent, Lausanne, Switzerland)	No	4.7 T	13
Mobin-Uddin IVC/umbrella filter (American Edwards, Santa Ana, CA)	No	4.7 T	13
New retrievable IVC filter (Thomas Jefferson University, Philadelphia, PA)	Yes	1.5 T	13
Palmaz endovascular stent (Ethicon, Somerville, NJ)	Yes	1.5 T	13
Prosthetic Ear Implants			
Cody tack	No	0.6 T	8
Cochlear implant (3M/House)	Yes	0.6 T	8
Cochlear implant (3M/Vienna)	Yes	0.6 T	8
House-type incus prosthesis	No	0.6 T	8
McGee stainless steel piston	No	0.6 T	8
Reuter drain tube	No	0.6 T	6
Richards House-type wire loop (Richard's Company, Nashville, TN)	No	1.5 T	1
Richards-McGee Piston (Richard's Company, Nashville, TN)	No	1.5 T	1
Richards Plasti-pore with Armstrong-style platinum ribbon (Richard's Company, Nashville, TN)	No	1.5 T	1
Richards-Schuknecht Teflon-wire (Richard's Company, Nashville, TN)	No	1.5 T	1
Richard Trapeze platinum ribbon (Richard's Company, Nashville, TN)	No	1.5 T	1
Shuknecht Gelfoam and wire prosthesis, Armstrong-style (Richard's Company, Nashville, TN)	No	1.5 T	6
Shea stainless steel and teflon wire prosthesis	No	1.5 T	6
Xomed stapes prosthesis Robinson-style (Richard's Company, Nashville, TN)	No	1.5 T	1

Contd...

Contd...

Metallic Implant or Object	*Deflection*	*Highest Field Strength*	*Reference*
Prosthetic Heart Valves			
Beall (Coratomic Inc., Indiana, PA)	Yes*	2.35 T	12
Bjork-Shiley (convexo/concave) (Shiley Inc., Irvine CA)	No	1.5 T	11
Bjork-Shiley (universal/spherical) (Shiley Inc., Irvine CA)	Yes*	1.5 T	11
Bjork-Shiley, Model MBC (Shiley Inc., Irvine CA)	Yes*	2.35 T	5
Bjork-Shiley, Model 25 MBRC 11030 (Shiley Inc., Irvine CA)	Yes*	2.35 T	5
Carpentier-Edwards, Model 2650 (American Edwards Laboratories, Santa Ana, CA)	Yes*	2.35 T	5
Carpentier-Edwards (porcine) (American Edwards Laboratories, Santa Ana, CA)	Yes*	2.35 T	12
Hall-Kaster, Model A7700 (Medtronic, Minneapolis, MN)	Yes*	1.5 T	11
Hancock I (porcine) (Johnson and Johnson, Anaheim, CA)	Yes*	1.5 T	11
Hancock II (porcine) (Johnson and Johnson, Anaheim, CA)	Yes*	1.5 T	11
Hancock extracorporeal, Model 242R (Johnson and Johnson, Anaheim, CA)	Yes*	2.35 T	5
Hancock extracorporeal, Model M 4365-33 (Johnson and Johnson, Anaheim, CA)	Yes*	2.35 T	5
Hancock Vascor, Model 505 (Johnson and Johnson, Anaheim, CA)	No	2.35 T	5
Ionescu-Shiley, (Universal ISM)	Yes*	2.35 T	5
Lillehi-Kaster, Model 300S (Medical Inc., Inver Grove Heights, MN)	Yes*	2.35 T	12
Lillehi-Kaster, Model 5009 (Medical Inc., Inver Grove Heights, MN)	Yes*	2.35 T	5

Contd...

Contd...

Metallic Implant or Object	*Deflection*	*Highest Field Strength*	*Reference*
Medtronic Hall (Medtronic Inc., Minneapolis, MN)	Yes*	2.35 T	12
Medtronic Hall, Model A7700-D-16 (Medtronic Inc., Minneapolis, MN)	Yes*	2.35 T	5
Omnicarbon, Model 3523T029 (Medical Inc., Inver Grove Heights, MN)	Yes*	2.35 T	5
Omniscience, Model 6522 (Medical Inc., Inver Grove Heights, MN)	Yes*	2.35 T	5
Smeloff-cutter (Cutter Laboratories, Berkeley, CA)	Yes*	2.35 T	5
Starr-Edwards, Model 1260 (American Edwards Laboratories, Santa Ana, CA)	Yes*	2.35 T	12
Starr-Edwards, Model 2320 (American Edwards Laboratories, Santa Ana, CA)	Yes*	2.35 T	12
Starr-Edwards, Model 2400 (American Edwards Laboratories, Santa Ana, CA)	No	1.5 T	11
Starr-Edwards, Model Pre 6000 (American Edwards Laboratories, Santa Ana, CA)	Yes	1.5 T	12
Starr-Edwards, Model 6520 (American Edwards Laboratories, Santa Ana, CA)	Yes*	2.35 T	5
St. Jude (St. Jude Medical Inc., St. Paul, MN)	No	1.5 T	11
St. Jude, Model A 101 (St. Jude Medical Inc., St. Paul, MN)	Yes*	2.35 T	5
St. Jude, Model M 101 (St. Jude Medical Inc., St. Paul, MN)	Yes*	2.35 T	5
Orthopedic Materials and Devices			
AML femoral component bipolar hip prosthesis (Zimmer, Warsaw, IN)	No	1.5 T	11

Contd...

Contd...

Metallic Implant or Object	*Deflection*	*Highest Field Strength*	*Reference*
Harris hip prosthesis (Zimmer, Warsaw, IN)	No	1.5 T	11
Jewett nail (Zimmer, Warsaw, IN)	No	1.5 T	11
Kirschner intermedullary rod (Kirschner Medical, Timonium, MD)	No	1.5 T	11
Stainless steel plate (Zimmer, Warsaw, IN)	No	1.5 T	11
Stainless steel screw (Zimmer, Warsaw, IN)	No	1.5 T	11
Stainless steel mesh (Zimmer, Warsaw, IN)	No	1.5 T	11
Stainless steel wire (Zimmer, Warsaw, IN)	No	1.5 T	11
Penile Implants			
Penile implant, AMS Malleable 600 (American Medical Systems, Minnetonka, MN)	No	1.5 T	10
Penile implant, AMS 700 CX Inflatable (American Medical Systems, Minnetonka, MN)	No	1.5 T	10
Penile implant, flexi-flate (Surgitek Medical Engineering Corp. Racine, WI)	No	1.5 T	10
Penile implant, flexi-rod (Standard) (Surgitek Medical Engineering Corp. Racine, WI)	No	1.5 T	10
Penile implant, flexi-rod II (Firm) (Surgitek, Medical Engineering Corp. Racine, WI)	No	1.5 T	10
Penile implant, Jonas (Dacomed Corp. Minneapolis, MN)	No	1.5 T	10
Penile implant, mentor flexible (Mentor Corp. Minneapolis, MN)	No	1.5 T	10

Contd...

Contd...

Metallic Implant or Object	*Deflection*	*Highest Field Strength*	*Reference*
Penile implant, mentor inflatable (Mentor Corp. Minneapolis, MN)	No	1.5 T	10
Penile implant, Omniphase (Dacomed Corp. Minneapolis, MN)	Yes	1.5 T	10
Miscellaneous Metallic Implants and Objects			
Artificial urinary sphincter, AMS 800 (American Medical Systems, Minnetonka, MN)	No	1.5 T	11
BB's (Daisy)	Yes	1.5 T	15
BB's (Crosman)	Yes	1.5 T	15
Cerebral ventricular shunt tube connector, Accu-flow, straight (Codman, Randolph, MA)	No	1.5 T	11
Cerebral ventricular shunt tube connector Accu-flow, right angle (Codman, Randolph, MA)	No	1.5 T	11
Cerebral ventricular shunt tube connector Accu-flow, T-connector (Codman, Randolph, MA)	No	1.5 T	11
Cerebral ventricular shunt tube connector (type unknown)	Yes	0.147 T	10
Contraceptive diaphragm, all flex (Ortho Pharmaceutical, Raritan, NJ)	Yes*	1.5 T	11
Contraceptive diaphragm, flat spring (Ortho Pharmaceutical, Raritan, NJ)	Yes*	1.5 T	11
Contraceptive diaphragm, koroflex (Young Drug Products, Piscataway, NJ)	Yes*	1.5T	11
Forceps (Titanium)	No	1.44 T	10
Hakim valve and pump	No	1.44 T	10

Contd...

Contd...

Metallic Implant or Object	*Deflection*	*Highest Field Strength*	*Reference*
Intraocular lens implant (Binkhorst, iridocapsular lense, platinum-iridium loop	No	1.0 T	3
Intraocular lens implant (Binkhorst, iridocapsular lens, titanium loop	No	1.0 T	3
Intraocular lens implant (Worst, platinum clip lens)	No	1.0 T	3
Intrauterine Contraceptive Device, (IUD), Copper T (Searle Pharmaceuticals, Chicago, IL)	No	1.5 T	7
Tantalum powder	No	1.44 T	9

(The "highest field strength" refers to the strongest static magnetic field that was used for the evaluation of the various metallic implant and objects. If no deflection was observed at low to midfield strengths, it is still possible for deflection to occur at higher static magnetic field strengths. Furthermore, if deflection was observed at low to midfield strengths, it will be greater at higher static megnetic fields).

*Denotes metallic implants or objects that were considered to be safe for MR imaging despite being deflected by the static magnetic field. For example, certain prosthetic heart valves were deflected by the static magnetic field but the actual force was considered to be less than the force exerted on the valves in an *in vivo* situation by the beating heart.[1,2] Refer to indicated reference for additional informationl. Manufacturer information provided if indicated in article or otherwise known. Note that, besides producing movement, the elctromagnetic fields used for MRI may produce other adverse effects in metallic bioimplants by inducing electrical current and/or heating. Although heating has not been evaluated for most of the bioimplants listed, data in the literature indicates that the heating of small implants and most larger ones is negligible during MRI.[3,4] There has been no report of electrical currents induced in metallic bioimplants. SS—stainless steel.

Courtesy from Shellock F

1. Shellock FG, Crues JV. High field strength MR imaging and metallic biomedical implants: An ex vivo evaluation of deflection forces. *AJR* 1988;151:811-814.
2. Soulen RL, Budinger TF, Higgins CB. Magnetic resonance imaging of prosthetic heart valves. *Radiology* 1985;154:705-707.
3. Davis PL, Crooks L, Arakawa M, McRee R, Kaufman L, Margulis AR. Potential hazards in NMR imaging: Heating effects of changing magnetic fields and RF fields on small metallic implants. *AJR* 1981;137:857-860.
4. Shellock FG, Crues JV. High field MR imaging of metallic biomedical implants: An in vitro evaluation of deflection forces and temperature induced in large prostheses (abstr). *Radiology* 1987;165:150.

Five

MRI—Pulse Sequences

INTRODUCTION

There are many different pulse sequences available, and each is designed for a specific purpose. The image weighting, contrast and quality is determined by the type of pulse sequence we use.

PULSE SEQUENCES

Types

1. Spin echo (SE) pulse sequences
   a. Conventional spin echo (CSE) pulse sequence
   b. Fast spin echo (FSE) pulse sequence
2. Inversion recovery (IR) pulse sequences
   a. STIR (short inversion recovery)
   b. FLAIR (fluid attenuated inversion recovery)
3. Gradient echo (GE) pulse sequences
   a. Coherent gradient echo pulse sequence
   b. Incoherent gradient echo pulse sequence
4. Steady state free precession (SSFP)
5. Ultrafast imaging
6. Echoplanar imaging

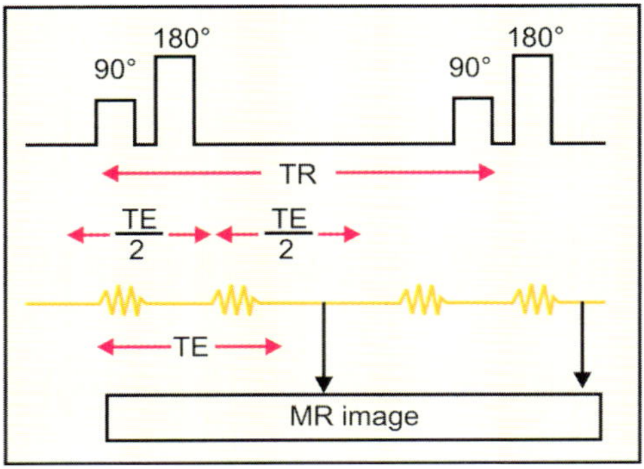

Fig. 5.1: Schematic illustration of a spin echo pulse sequence

Spin Echo (SE) Pulse Sequences (Fig. 5.1)

Conventional Spin Echo (CSE) Pulse Sequence

In this pulse sequence, a 90° excitation RF pulse is given followed by 180° rephasing RF pulse.

Uses

- These are the most commonly used pulse sequences
- May be used for almost every examination
- Produce optimum signal-to-noise ratio (SNR) and contrast-to-noise ratio (CNR)
- T1, T2 and proton density weighting is possible (Figs 5.2 and 5.3).

Advantages

- Good image quality
- True T2 weighting is possible.

Disadvantages

- Scan times are relatively long
- More RF power deposition in the body.

Parameters

- *For T1 weighting*
  TE = 10-20 ms
  TR = 300-600 ms
  Approx. scan time
  = 4-6 minutes
- *For T2 weighting*
  TE = 80 ms
  TR = 2000 ms
  Approx. scan time
  = 7-15 minutes
- *Proton density*
  TE = 20 ms
  TR = 2000 ms
  Approx. scan time = 7-15 minutes

Fast Spin Echo (FSE) Pulse Sequence

In this type of pulse sequence, 90° excitation RF pulse will be delivered followed by several 180° rephasing RF pulses. In conventional spin echo (CSE), only one line of K-space is filled per TR. So the CSE takes longer scan time. But in fast spin echo several lines of K-space will be filled per TR. Because of this reason, the scan times are reduced in fast spin echo. The number of lines of K-space filled per TR is referred to as Turbo Factor (tf) (or) echo train length (ETL). More the ETL, less the scan time (Fig. 5.4).

Uses

- Can be used as an alternative to spin echo
- Reduction in the scan time compared to conventional spin echo.

Advantages

- Scan times are greatly reduced
- High resolution matrices and multiple NEX can be used
- Improved image quality.

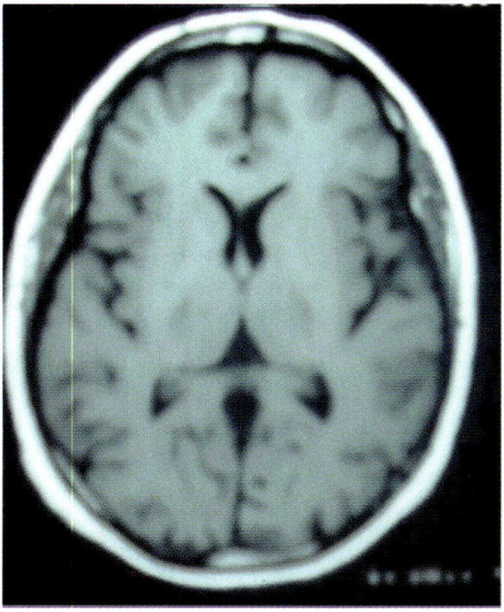

Fig. 5.2: Spin echo T1W1 CSF appears dark

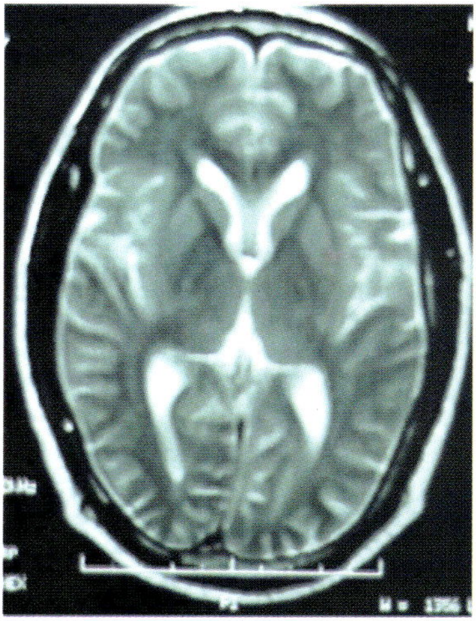

Fig. 5.3: Spin echo T2W1 CSF appears bright

Disadvantages

- Fat remains bright on T2 weighted images
- Image blurring may result

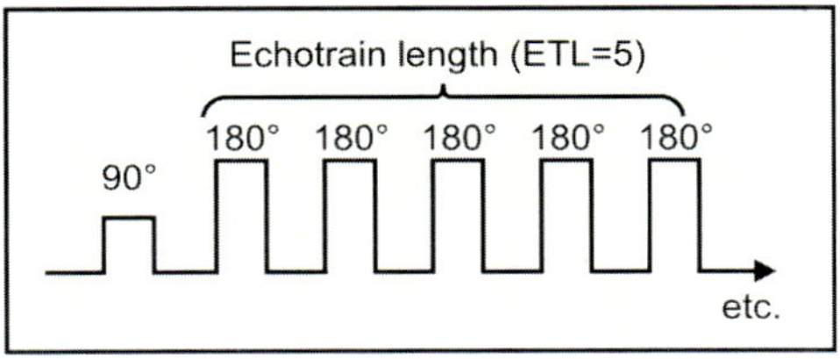

Fig. 5.4: Schematic illustration of fast spin echo

Parameters

- *T1 weighting*
  TE = 10-20 ms
  TR = 300-600 ms
  ETL = 2-6
  Approx. scan time = 30 sec to 60 sec/acq
- *T2 weighting*
  TE = 100 ms
  TR = 5000 ms
  ETL = 8-20
  Approx. scan time = 2 minutes

Proton Density Weighting

TE = 20 ms
TR = 3000 ms
Approx. scan time = 3-4 minutes

Inversion Recovery (IR) Pulse Sequences

These pulse sequences use 180° inverting RF pulse followed by 90° excitation RF pulse after certain time [Inversion Time (IT) or Time from Inversion (TI)].

Depending on the TI value, we can classify the IR sequences into:

1. Short inversion recovery (STIR)
2. Fluid attenuated inversion recovery (FLAIR)

If we apply 180° inverting RF pulse, the NMV (net magnetic vector) will be inverted through 180° into full saturation. When we remove the inverting pulse, the NMV

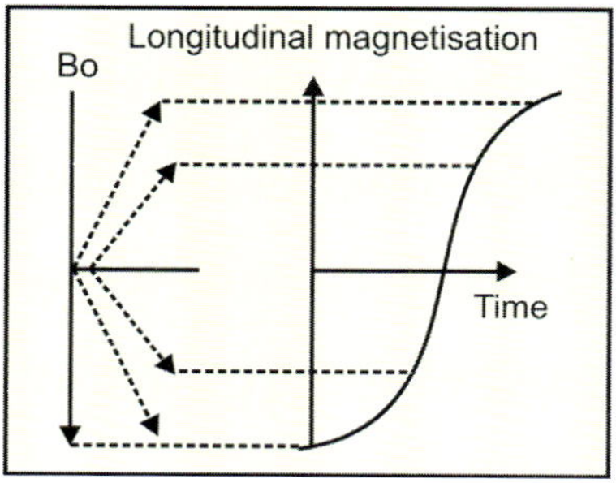

Fig. 5.5: Recovery from inversion

begins to relax back to Bo (static external magnetic field) (Fig. 5.5).

A 90° excitation pulse is then applied at a time from the 180° inverting pulse known as the TI time (Time from Inversion). The contrast of the image depends on the TI value (Fig. 5.6).

These sequences are used to generate heavily T1 weighted images bringing large difference between fat and water.

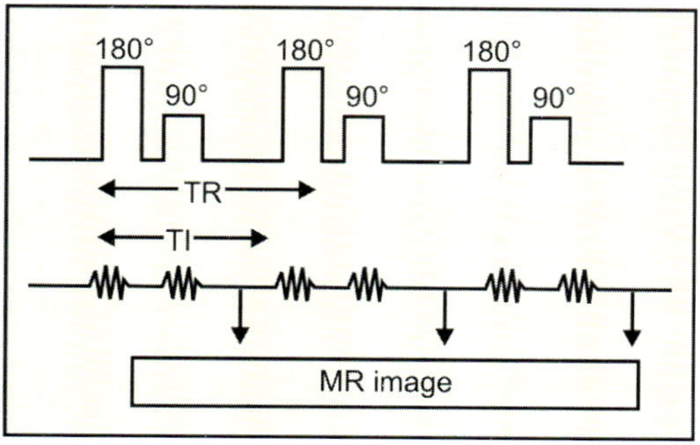

Fig. 5.6: Schematic illustration of the inversion recovery (IR) pulse sequence

Advantages

- Produces heavily T1 weighted images
- Very good signal-to-noise ratio (SNR).

Disadvantage

- Long scan times.

STIR (Short Inversion Recovery) Pulse Sequence

This sequence is used to suppress the fat signal from the anatomy of interest. Here we use a TI value that corresponds to the time it takes fat to recover from full inversion to the transverse plane so that there is no longitudinal magnetization corresponding to fat. When the 90° RF excitation pulse is applied, the fat is flipped 90° to 180°, so there will not be any fat signal. It will suppress the fat in STIR. Generally, a TI value of around 100-200 ms is used. This TI value may slightly vary depending on the field strength (Fig. 5.7, Table 5.1).

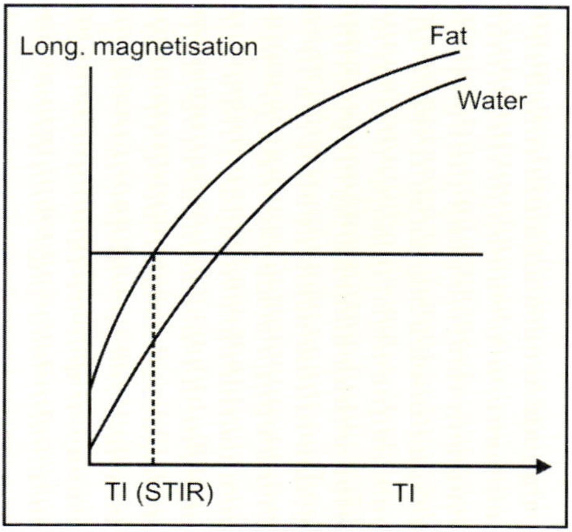

Fig. 5.7: T1 determination of STIR

Table 5.1: Optimal inversion times for a given field strength (for STIR)

Field strength (T)	*TI (ms)*
1.5	120-150
1.0	100-230
0.5	90-115
0.2	75-90

Uses

- Used to suppress the fat signal in T1 weighted image.

Disadvantage Should not be used with contrast enhancement.

Parameters

TE = 10-30 ms
TR = 2000 ms
TI = 150-200 ms
Average scan time = 5-15 minutes.

FLAIR (Fluid Attenuated Inversion Recovery)

It is another variation in the IR pulse sequence which uses a TI value around 2000 ms. Usually, this sequence is used to suppress the signal from CSF containing areas.

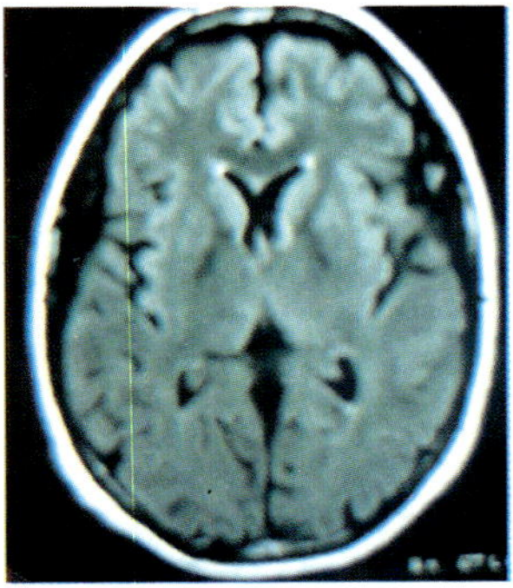

Fig. 5.8: FLAIR image (CSF appears more dark since it is heavily T1 weighted image)

Parameters

TE = Short or long depending on weighting

TR = 6000-8000 ms

TI = 2000 ms

Average scan time = 13-20 minutes

Gradient Echo (GE) Pulse Sequences

These sequences use variable flip angles and lesser repetition time (TR). The gradients are used to rephase the protons. We can apply the gradients quickly to rephase the protons (unlike 180° rephasing pulses in spin echo which takes some time to apply) (Figs 5.8 and 5.9).

Because of the quicker application of gradients and reduced repetition time and smaller flip angles, the scan times are greatly reduced in gradient echo pulse sequences. With this sequence, we can get T1 weighting, proton density weighting and $T2^*$ weighting.

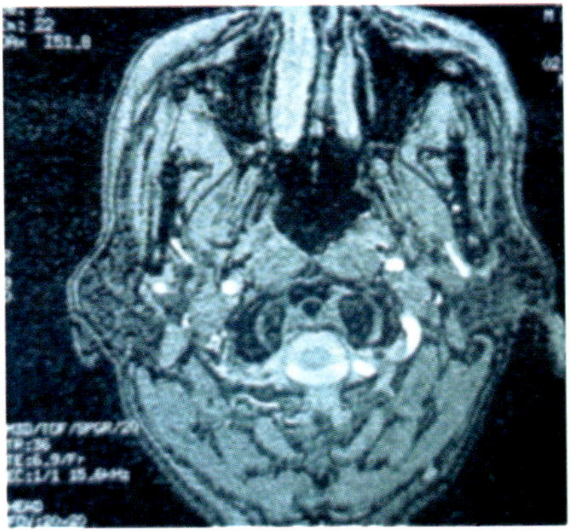

Fig. 5.9: Image obtained with gradient echo pulse sequence. Blood vessels appear bright on gradient echo pulse sequences

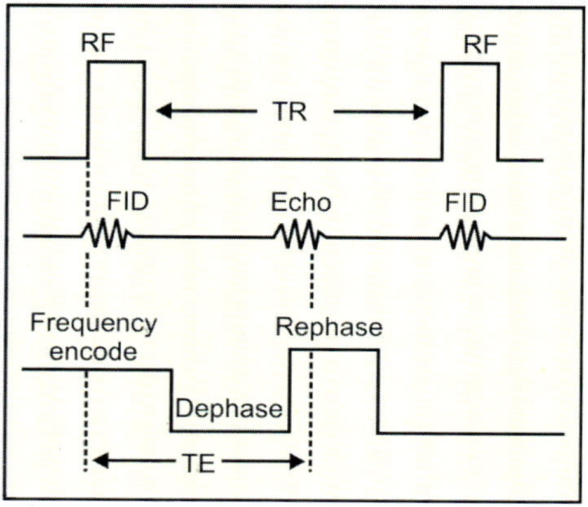

Fig. 5.10: Schematic illustration of gradient echo pulse sequence

Since the gradient does not compensate for magnetic field inhomogeneities, we will get T2* weighting (Fig. 5.10).

Uses

- Can be used to produce T1, proton density and T2* weighting
- Very minimal scan times
- Can be used for single slice breathhold acquisitions in abdomen and dynamic contrast enhancement
- Since these sequences are flow sensitive, can be used for MR angiography/MR myelography
- Less RF deposition into the body, i.e. less specific absorption rate (SAR).

Disadvantages

- Less signal-to-noise ratio when compared to SE pulse sequences

- True T2 weighting is not possible ($T2^*$ contrast rather than true T2)
- More work for the gradients
- More noise to the patient.

Steady State

In this state, the selected TR will be shorter than the T1 and T2 times of the tissues. In this state, there will be coexis-tence of both longitudinal and transverse magnetization. Most gradient echo sequences use the steady state. Generally, flip angles of 30° to 45° with TR of 20 to 50 ms favours the steady state.

Depending on the residual transverse magnetization in phase (or) out of phase GE pulse sequences are classified into:

1. Coherent (in phase) gradient echo pulse sequence
2. Incoherent (out of phase) gradient echo pulse sequence.

Coherent (in phase) Gradient Echo Pulse Sequences

These sequences use a variable flip angle excitation pulse followed by a frequency encoding gradient rephasing to produce a gradient echo. Here the steady state is maintained by selecting a TR shorter than the T1 and T2 times of the tissues. In this sequence, the tissue with long T2 values appear with high signal intensity.

Uses

- Increased $T2^*$ Dependence
- Very fast scans

- Preserves the transverse signal
- Good for angiography
- Can be acquired in a volume acquisition.

Disadvantages

- More gradient noise to the patient
- Poor SNR in 2D acquisitions compared to spin echo
- More magnetic susceptibility.

Parameters

- To maintain the steady state:
  - Flip angle: 30°-45°
  - TR-20-50 ms
- To maximize T2*
  - TE = 15-25 ms

Incoherent (Spoiled) Gradient Echo Pulse Sequences

These pulse sequences begin with a variable flip angle excitation pulse and use frequency encoding gradient rephasing to give a gradient echo. These sequences spoil (or) dephase the residual transverse magnetization so that its effect on image contrast is minimal.

Uses

- Increased T1 weighting
- Spoils the transverse signal
- Only the longitudinal signal contributes to the next RF pulse
- Good SNR in volume acquisition
- Can be acquired in 2D (or) volume
- Breath holding is possible.

Disadvantages

- Decreased SNR in 2D
- Loud gradient noise.

Parameters

- To maintain the steady state
  - Flip angle: 30°-45°
  - TR = 20-50 ms
- To maximize T1
  - TE = 5-10 ms is used.

Steady State Free Precession (SSFP)

These sequences are used to attain more T2 weighting. In this sequence the steady state is maintained.

Parameters

—Flip angle: 30°-45°
—TR = 20-50 ms

Advantages

- True T2 weighting is achieved
- Can be acquired in volume or 2D

Disadvantages

- Loud gradient noise
- Poor image quality

Ultrafast Sequences

- These sequences use coherent (or) incoherent gradient echo pulse sequences
- Only a portion of the RF pulse is used
- Only a portion of the echo is read

Because of the above reasons, the scan time is drastically reduced.

Echoplanar Imaging (EPI)

- The fastest scan acquisition modes in MRI are the EPI and the gradient echo pulse sequences.
- In echoplanar imaging all the lines of K-space will be filled in one shot. This is called single shot EPI (SS-EPI).
- If the echoes are generated by multiple 180° pulses, this is termed as spin echo echoplanar imaging (SE-EPI).
- If the gradients are used for the purpose of rephasing in EPI, then this sequence is called GE-EPI.
- GE-EPI and SS-EPI are faster than SE-EPI.
- SS-EPI sequences are more prone to artifacts such as chemical shift, distortion and blurring.
- In EPI the image may contain more $T2^*$ weighting which can be minimized by using 180° inverting pulse before excitation pulse.

Uses

- Improved cardiac and abdominal imaging
- Used in perfusion weighted imaging
- Useful in real time and interventional MR-guided procedures.

PERFUSION WEIGHTED IMAGING (PWI)

This is a type of dynamic MR imaging by using GRE (or) EPI sequences with contrast enhancement to study the uptake of contrast medium by the lesion. This technique can be used in abnormalities of brain, pancreas, liver and prostate.

DIFFUSION WEIGHTED IMAGING (DWI)

In this type of MR imaging either GRE (or) EPI sequences are used to demonstrate the areas with restricted diffusion of extracellular water such as infarcted tissue. High signal intensity appears at the area of restricted diffusion. DWI is mainly useful in brain to differentiate salvageable and nonsalvageable tissue after brain stroke.

FUNCTIONAL MRI (FMRI)

It is a dynamic MR imaging Technique that acquires images of the brain during stimulus and also at rest. Then the two sets of images are subtracted to demonstrate functional brain activity. This technique is called BOLD (blood oxygenation level dependent). At the activated areas of brain, there will be increased signal intensity. fMRI is useful in evaluating the brain activity in the disorders of epilepsy, stroke and behavioural problems.

MAGNETIZATION TRANSFER (MT) CONTRAST

This is a technique used to suppress the background tissue thereby increasing the conspicuity of vessels and certain disease processes. MT contrast is useful in diagnosing hemorrhage, AIDS, multiple sclerosis and also to improve contrast in TOF-MRA images by suppressing background tissue.

MAGNETIC RESONANCE ANGIOGRAPHY (MRA)

MRA is a technique which allows us to acquire the images with high signal from flowing nuclei and low signal from stationary nuclei. This technique will allow us to see the blood vessels more clearly than surrounding. Generally, GRE pulse sequences are used to show flowing vessels as bright. There are two types of MRA techniques available.

They are: 1) Time of flight (TOF-MRA and 2) Phase-contrast MRA (PC-MRA).

Time of Flight MRA (TOF-MRA)

This technique commonly uses incoherent GRE pulse sequences in conjunction with TR and flip angle combinations that saturate background tissue but allowing moving spins to show high signal intensity. This technique is used in demonstrating arterial and venous flow in head, neck and peripheral vessels.

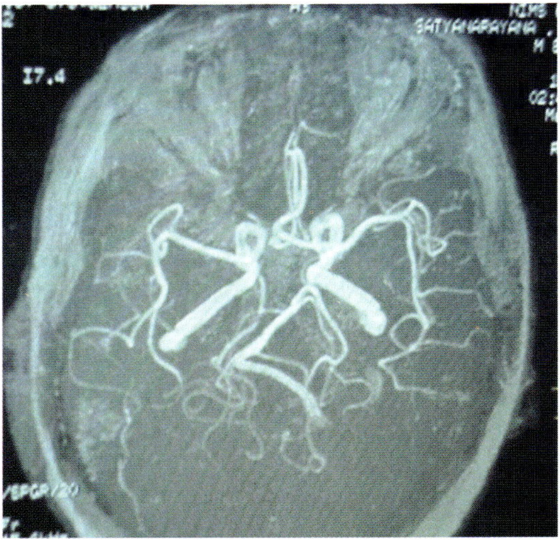

Fig. 5.11: 3D TOF MRA showing intracranial vessels

Phase Contrast MRA (PC-MRA)

This technique usually uses coherent GRE sequences. It provides excellent background suppression. But the scan

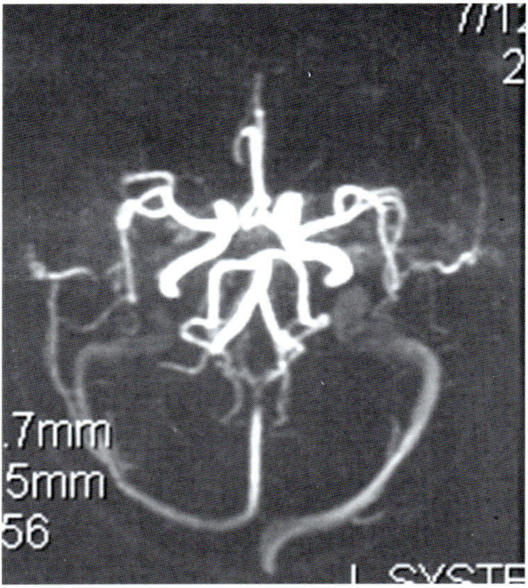

Fig. 5.12: 3D PC-MRA image

times with PC-MRA are longer than the scan times of GE pulse sequences are flow sensitive hence used for MRA (magnetic resonance angiography).

ACRONYMS USED BY MANUFACTURERS (Table 5.2)

Table 5.2: A comparison of the acronyms used by manufacturers

	GE	*Philips*	*Siemens*
Spin echo	MEMP VEMP	Spin echo	Spin echo
Fast spin echo	FSE	TSE	TSE
Coherent gradient echo	GRASS	FFE	FISP
Incoherent gradient echo (RF spoiled)	SPGR	T1 FFE	
Incoherent gradient echo (gradient spoiled)	MPGR		FLASH
Steady state free precession	SSFP	T2 FFE	PSIF
Inversion recovery	MPIR	IR	IR
Short T1 inversion recovery	STIR	SPIR	STIR
Ultrafast	Fast GRASS SPGR (IR/DE PREP)	TFE FLASH 3D MP RAGE	Turbo
Presaturation	SAT	REST	SAT
Gradient moment rephasing	Flow comp	FLAG	Resp. trigger
Signal averaging	NEX	NSA	AC
Partial averaging	Fractional NEX	Half scan	Half fourier
Partial echo	Fractional echo	Partial echo	
No phase wrap	No phase wrap	Fold over suppression	Over sampling

Contd..

Contd..

	GE	*Philips*	*Siemens*
Rectangular FOV	Rect FOV	Rect FOV	Half Fourier imaging

Abbreviations used in Table

AC	:	Number of acquisitions
FSE	:	Fast spin echo
FFE	:	Fast field echo
FLAG	:	Flow adjusted gradients
FISP	:	Fast imaging with steady precession
FLASH	:	Fast low angled shot
FAST	:	Fourier acquired steady state technique
GMR	:	Gradient movement rephasing
IR	:	Inversion recovery
MPGR	:	Multi planar gradient recalled acquisition in the steady state
MPIR	:	Multiplanar inversion recovery
NEX	:	Number of excitations
NSA	:	Number of signal averages
PSIF	:	Mirrored FISP
REST	:	Regional saturation technique
SPGR	:	Spoiled gradient recalled acquisition in the steady state
STIR	:	Short T1 inversion recovery
SPIR	:	Spectrally selective inversion recovery
SAT	:	Saturation
TFE	:	Turbo field echo
TSE	:	Turbo spin echo

Six

Tissue Characteristics

Magnetic resonance imaging is a diagnostic modality providing cross-sectional imaging of the entire body in any plane with no radiation risk to the patient. There are no known adverse effects.

ROLE OF MRI IN DISEASES

MRI has unique properties. It is a complex yet interesting imaging technique utilized for the diagnosis of various diseases in all parts of the body. MRI is very sensitive to certain pathologies, demonstrating disorders not shown on other imaging modalities, i.e. CT. The rapid advances in MRI have resulted in many new pulse sequences providing details about tissue characterization.

Production of Image

When the patient is placed in the scanner, the applied external magnetic field (EMF) induces a net nuclear magnetization (NNM) in the longitudinal axis of the patient. This NNM is rotated through 90 degrees by the RF pulse. When the RF pulse is discontinued, relaxation back to the original state occurs, i.e. recovery of the magnetization in the longitudinal plane and decay of magnetization in the transverse plane. The recovery of longitudinal magnetization is known as spin lattice or T1 recovery. The decay of transverse magnetization is known as spin spin relaxation or T2 decay. T1 is determined by how quickly the nuclei can transfer energy to their surrounding environment (lattice) and return to a lower energy state. T2 is determined by how quickly the nuclei can exchange energy with neighboring nuclei to produce random distribution of the precessing nuclei about the magnetic field.

The sensitivity of MRI to certain substances, i.e. water and iron compounds, is of particular importance in clinical imaging. For example, the high sensitivity of MRI to tissue water allows the effective demonstration of brain edema. All types of edema namely vasogenic, cytotoxic and interstitial, result in altered signals and are best seen on T2 weighted images as a bright signal.

The marked differences in the relaxation times of water and brain tissue enable the differentiation of tissues. For example, smaller structures such as cranial nerves that are bathed in cerebrospinal fluid (CSF) are well demonstrated on MRI. MRI is superior in the demonstration of tumors and other abnormalities of nerves, i.e. acoustic neuromas and lesions involving the optic chiasma.

The sensitivity of MRI to paramagnetic substances such as iron is of great clinical importance, as lesions of increased iron in pallideus, substantia nigra, red nucleus and dentate nucleus demonstrate a low signal on T2 weighted images.

MRI is sensitive for the detection of cerebral ischemia, plus has the advantage of evaluating subacute and chronic trauma cases.

Advantages of Magnetic Resonance Imaging

1. Nonionising radiation
2. No known biological hazards
3. Multiplanar imaging: images can be obtained in all planes namely coronal, sagittal, axial or any oblique plane
4. High soft tissue resolution
5. Superior soft tissue characterization when compared to CT as the tissue is studied in T1, T2 and other sequences
6. Blood flow imaging
7. Non-invasive imaging technique.

Disadvantages

1. High cost
2. Claustrophobia (fear of enclosed spaces). The wider bore design associated with present equipment has resulted in a reduction in the occurrence of MRI induced claustrophobia
3. Longer imaging time: difficult to image critically ill and very uncooperative patients
4. Cortical bone and calcific lesions are poorly visualized
5. High degree of technical expertise is required
6. Patients with pacemakers, surgical clips, otologic and ocular implants, etc. are unable to undergo an MRI examination.

MRI Image

The image represents a display of the MR signal. The signal intensity depends on both the tissue and equipment (operator) parameters. It is important to understand that the gray scale on a MR image is not readily predictable and can be dramatically altered by machine-dependent parameters such as choice of pulse sequence, time between pulses (TE), repetition time (TR), inversion time (TI) etc. There are four main tissue MR parameters contributing to the signal intensity of an image: i) proton density, ii) T1, iii) T2 and iv) blood flow.

The MR image depends on the following four main factors;

- T1 relaxation time
- T2 decay time
- Proton density
- Blood flow.

Proton (Spin) Density, T1W and T2W

MR imaging is related to the density of mobile protons. Proton density is represented by the symbol (PD). The PD image is obtained using a spin echo sequence with long TR and short TE or a gradient echo sequence with a low flip angle. As the PD of various tissue obtained differs only by a few percent, this pulse sequence is not widely used.

Air contains a low density of protons; therefore sinuses show no proton image. Trabecular bone, on the other hand, contains many protons but still generates no signal. This is because the protons are tightly bound and have a T2 decay time so small that the signals vanish before conventional MR imaging is able to detect them.

Relaxation times are affected by the chemical composition of the tissue being studied. Each normal tissue in the body has a specific relaxation time which is either shortened or prolonged by certain pathological changes.

The choice of a short TR enhances the T1 contrast between fats and liquids. On the T2 decay curve, each tissue starts at a different level. Fats are characterized by a short T2 and liquids by a long T2: there is a crossing point between the two curves where the two substances show an isointense signal.

INTENSITIES OF NORMAL ANATOMICAL STRUCTURES

Normal anatomical structures are listed below according to their signal intensity on T1 weighted images (Table 6.1).

1. High intensity
   - Fat
     - Orbital
     - Scalp

Table 6.1: Typical values for normal and some abnormal tissues at 1.0 T

Tissue type	*Relative proton density*	*T1 (ms)*	*T2 (ms)*
Lipids	0.6	250	50
White matter	0.75	670	85
Gray matter	0.85	920	95
Peripheral muscle	0.8	620	45
Liver	0.70	570	45
Cerebrospinal fluid	1	2000	1000
Edema	0.90	1060	150
Brain tumor	0.90	1410	200
MS plaque	0.90	1100	150

- Mucous
- Marrow
  - Cranium
  - Sphenoid, clivus
  - Vertebra
- Cartilage of nasal septum

2. Low intensity

- Venous sinuses
- Veins
  - Internal jugular
  - Superior ophthalmic
  - Internal cerebral
  - Vein of Galen
- Cortical veins
- Arteries
  - Carotid
  - Ophthalmic
  - Anterior, middle and posterior cerebral
  - Anterior inferior cerebellar artery (AICA)
  - Posterior inferior cerebellar artery (PICA)
  - Vertebral-basilar
- Paranasal sinuses
- Choroid plexus
- Cortical bone
- Falx cerebri
- Tentorium
- Calcified cartilage
- Calcified structures, e.g. pineal gland.

When excited protons return to equilibrium, they relax inducing a signal. The combined signal generates the MR image.

Table 6.2: High and low MR signals

	High MR signal (White)	*Low MR signal (Black)*
Proton density	High	Low
T1 relaxation	Short	Long
T2 relaxation	Long	Short
Blood flow	Slow/stationary	Fast/turbulent

If the emitted signal is low, it is termed hypointense and represented in black. If the emitted signal is high, it is termed hyperintense and represented in white.

- **T1 weighted images (Fig. 6.1):**
  Hypointense: tissue with a long T1
  Hyperintense: tissue with a short T2

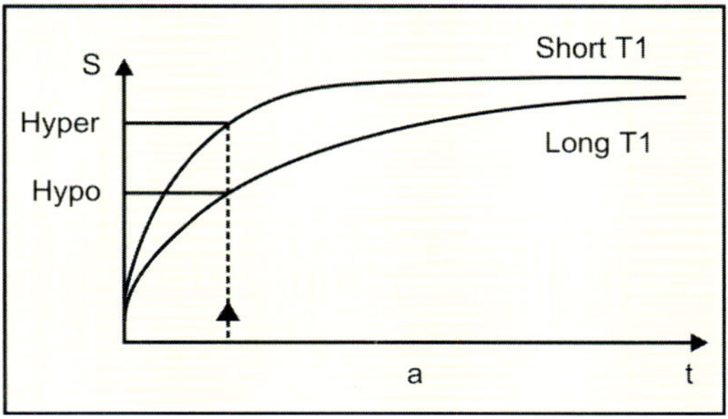

Fig. 6.1: T1 characteristics of body tissues

- **T2 weighted images (Fig. 6.2):**
  Hypointense: tissue with a short T2
  Hyperintense: tissue with a long T2

Liquid produces a hypointense signal on a T1 weighted pulse sequence and a hyperintense signal on a T2 weighted pulse sequence. Fat, on the contrary, has an opposite signal, i.e. hyperintense on a T1 pulse sequence and hypointense

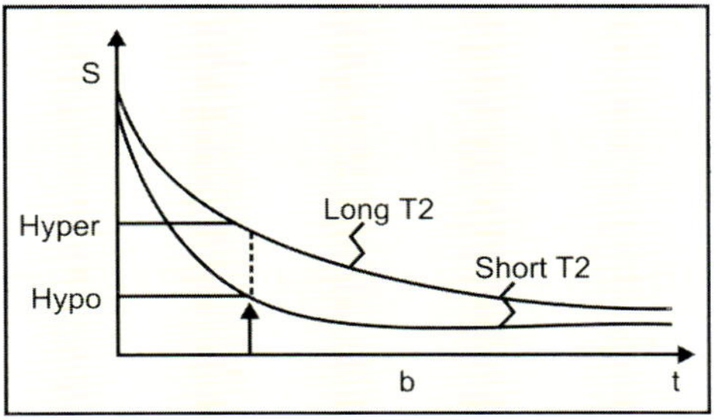

Fig. 6.2: T2 characteristics of body tissues

on a T2 weighted pulse sequence. Both fat and water have the same signal (isosignal) in a mixed pulse sequence (Figs 6.3 and 6.4).

Causes of hypointensity (on short flip angle, long TE gradient echo images):

- Hemorrhage
  - Deoxyhemoglobin
  - Ferritin/hemosiderin
  - Other iron forms
- Calcification
  - Diamagnetic calcium salts
  - Associated paramagnetic ions
- Air containing paranasal sinuses
- Normal brain iron
- Paramagnetic contrast agents
- Ferromagnetic devices, foreign bodies
- Intravascular deoxygenated blood.

***Pathological changes influencing image appearance*:**

Edema: Both cytotoxic edema and vasogenic edema are hypointense on T1 and hyperintense on T2 weighted pulse sequences. Necrosis, also appears hypointense on T1 and hyperintense on T2 weighted pulse sequences.

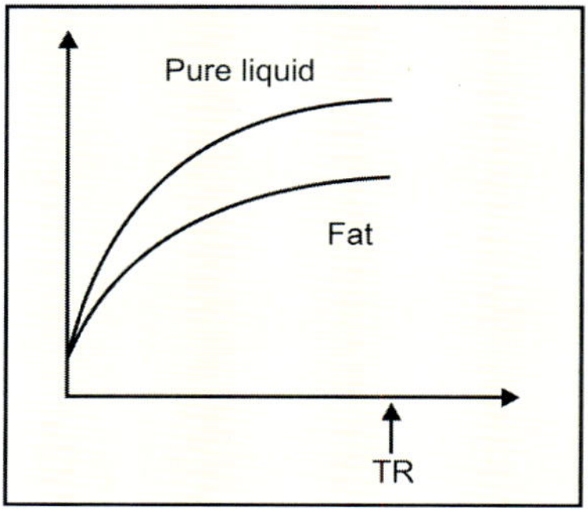

Fig. 6.3: Mixed sequence with short TR

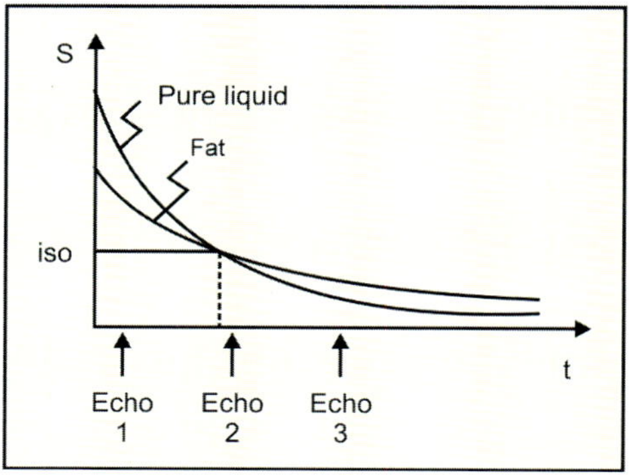

Fig. 6.4: Mixed sequence with three echoes

Gliosis: On T2 weighted pulse sequences, gliosis appears as distinct areas of high signal intensity.

Radiation effects: Radiation may cause a decrease in signal intensity on T2 weighted pulse sequences.

Cysts: Cysts are hypointense on T1 and hyperintense on T2 weighted pulse sequences and are similar to CSF in intensity.

Demyelination: Areas of demyelination are visualized as hyperintense signals on T2 weighted pulse sequences.

Fatty changes: Increased fat or lipid content as in epidermoid tumors, result in a characteristic high intensity lesion on T1 weighted pulse sequences.

Fibrosis: Fibrosis, seen in postoperative disk surgery, appears hypointense on both T1 and T2 weighted pulse sequences.

Gray-white Matter

The T2 of white matter (WM) is less than the T2 of gray matter (GM) and the T1 of WM is less than the T1 of GM. As WM has a shorter T1 and T2, it appears brighter on T1 weighted images whilst the short T2 makes it appear less bright on T2 weighted images. The brightness of WM on T1 weighted images is attributed to the membrane lipid myelin in the brain.

Vascular Structures

If hydrogen passes through the image volume faster than the time taken to perform an imaging sequence, there will be no detectable signal. The signal intensity of flowing blood is a function of the percentage of moving hydrogen nuclei, their velocity and the temporal parameters of the imaging technique. The normal carotid artery, basilar artery and venous sinuses have no detectable signal, appearing black on MR images.

Intravascular blood appears either white or black on MR images depending on its velocity of flow or turbulence: fast flowing blood appears black, whilst slow flowing blood appears white.

Short T1 (White)	Retro-orbital fat
	White matter
	Internal capsule
	Thalamus
	Cerebellar gray matter
	Caudate nucleus
	Cortical gray matter
	Cerebrospinal fluid
Long T1 (Black)	Ocular vitreous
Long T2 (White)	Cerebrospinal fluid
	Ocular vitreous
	Cortical gray matter
	Cerebellar gray matter
	Caudate nucleus
	Orbital fat
	Cortical white matter
Short T2 (Black)	Internal capsule
High proton density (White)	Fat
	Cortical gray matter
	Cerebellar gray matter
	Caudate
	Cortical white matter
	Internal capsule
	CSF
	Bone
Low proton density (Black)	Air

Pathological Changes and Effect of Relaxation Time

Both the T1 and T2 recovery times can either be shortened or prolonged by the following;

T1 Shortened

- Lipid
- Paramagnetic substance:
  a. Copper
  b. Iron
  c. Manganese
- Mucus
- Cholesterol
- Postradiation changes (after two weeks)
- Hemorrhage (methemoglobin)
- Increased protein content
- Melanin

T2 Shortened

- Air
- Calcium
- Cortical bone
- Paramagnetic substances
- Fat

T1 Prolonged

- Air
- Calcium
- Cortical bone
- Edema
- Demyelination
- Neoplasia

- Infection
- Ischemia
- Infarction
- CSF

T2 Prolonged

- Demyelination
- Infection
- CSF
- Ischemia
- Neoplasia
- Edema

Appearance of Blood on MR Images Utilizing Various Imaging Techniques

Bright

- Gradient echo pulse sequences
- Flow compensation (slow flow)
- Short echo time
- Thin two-dimensional gradient echo section oriented perpendicular to direction of blood flow
- MR contrast agents shorten the T1 relaxation time of blood
- Spiral scan pulse sequence
- Segmented turbo flash pulse sequence.

Dark

- Spin echo
- Presaturation pulse
- Long echo time
- Thin two-dimensional spin echo or fast spin echo sections oriented perpendicular to direction of flow

- Super paramagnetic iron oxide to shorten T2 relaxation time of blood.

Thrombosis and clot formation are complex dynamic processes. Clot retraction, cellular infiltration, fibrinolysis, red blood cell morphology, hemoglobin desaturation and the development of blood degradation products interact to affect the MR appearance (Table 6.3).

Table 6.3: MR appearance of hemorrhage

Hemoglobin stage	*MR signal*	*RBC morphology*
1. Oxyhemoglobin	Center, hyperintense thin peripheral rim surrounding edema	Normal
2. Deoxyhemoglobin	Isointense	Spherocytes
3. Methemoglobin	Hypointense	Echinocytes
4. Macrophages with hemosiderin and ferritin	Hyperintense Blooming of dark signal	Dehydrated Lysed

Extrinsic factors such as field strength and pulse sequences also affect the MR signal.

Hyperacute Clots and Oxyhemoglobin

Oxyhemoglobin (OxyHb) is present in hyperacute clots for only a few minutes or up to a few hours. OxyHb contains ferrous iron, lacks unpaired electrons and is diamagnetic. Therefore, OxyHb does not affect T1 and T2 relaxation times. The MR signal of hyperacute hematoma can be attributed to its protein traces containing water content. Hyperacute clots are typically isointense with GM on T1 weighted images and hyperintense on T2 weighted images.

Acute Clots and Deoxyhemoglobin

Hemoglobin desaturation from oxyHb to deoxyhemoglobin (DeoxyHb) occurs within a few hours of hemoglobin. As

DeoxyHb contains ferrous iron with four unpaired electrons in a high spin state, it is strongly paramagnetic. DeoxyHb lacks the ability to cause proton electron dipoledipole (PEDD), proton relaxation enhancement and T1 shortening, appearing isointense with brain parenchyma on T1 weighted images.

If DeoxyHb is sequestrated within RBCs, as water diffuses freely across the cell membrane, it experiences a substantial magnetic susceptibility gradient. This results is phase dispersion and subsequent preferential T2 proton relaxation enhancement (T2-PRE).

The susceptibility effects seen with acute clots become more pronounced with progressive T2 weighting. Acute clots with DeoxyHb typically appear moderately hypointense on balanced (long TR/short TE) pulse sequences and profoundly hypointense on T2 weighted or gradient refocused pulse sequences.

Subacute Clots and Methemoglobin

Methemoglobin (MetHb) is present in subacute hematoma and can be seen from a few days to a few months following hemorrhage. MetHb is ferric, has five unpaired electrons and is strongly paramagnetic.

Early subacute hematomas have a bright signal on T1 weighted images. The bright signal typically begins at the hematoma periphery and progresses inwards. Thus, the center of early subacute clots remains relatively isointense on T1 weighted images and the rim becomes hyperintense. In the early subacute stage of hematoma formation, MetHb is contained within intact RBCs and preferentially increases T2-PRE. This T2 shortening results in low signal on long TR/short TE, i.e. proton density weighted pulse sequences.

Early subacute clots are profoundly hypointense on T2 weighted and gradient refocused pulse sequences.

In the late subacute stage, hemolysis results in the accumulation of extracellular MetHb within the hematoma cavity. MetHB in a free solution is extremely hyperintense on T1 and T2 weighted images.

Chronic Clots and Iron Storage

In the early chronic stage, a pool of dilute-free MetHb is surrounded by the ferritin and hemosiderin containing vascularized wall. At this stage, clots are typically homogeneously hyperintense on both T1 and T2 weighted images, with a pronounced hypointense signal rim on T2 weighted images. Edema and mass effect diminish and then disappear.

The long-term residue of late chronic hematomas following brain hemorrhage persists as macrophages laden with iron storage products remain around the margins old clots for years. Two substances are present in the late phase of resolving cerebral hematomas namely ferritin and hemosiderin.

Hemosiderin is isointense on T1 and extremely hypointense on T2 weighted images. Due to strong magnetic susceptibility effects, ferritin and hemosiderin appear profoundly hypointense on gradient echo pulse sequences.

CLINICAL APPLICATIONS

MRI of Brain and Spine

Brain

Tumors

Although results have proved to be disappointing, especially in the detection of small calcifications, MRI, is at present superior to CT in its ability to detect tumor. In comparison with CT, MRI has the advantage of detecting lesions in the posterior fossa, at the edge of calvanium and is superior for lesions near the base of the skull and the pituitary fossa. MRI has the added advantage of characterizing tissue better in tumors with lipomatous component and in tumors appearing as enhancing foci not distinguishable from vascular structures on CT.

Hemorrhage–Ischemic Stroke

Both these condition are easily detected by MRI. For example, the detection of thrombosis/stenosis is a very promising application of MR angiography. It is also possible to separate the hemorrhagic and edematous component of an infarct. Using special pulse sequences, i.e. diffusion imaging, a stroke can be detected at the onset of ischemia.

Trauma

In comparison with CT, MRI has the advantage of demonstrating the entire extent of the extracerebral collection plus superior evaluation of diffuse axonal injury and sequelae of trauma. An added advantage of MRI when scanning trauma cases is its multiplanar capabilities, i.e. the ability to scan in different planes without moving the patient. Disadvantages include the longer scanning times and the inability to demonstrate the bony cranium.

Degenerative Diseases

MRI is extremely effective in diagnosing multiple sclerosis, subcortical arteriosclerotic encephalopathy, gliosis and syrinx. In the detection of demyelinating diseases, MRI is clearly superior to CT.

From the above, MRI is proving to be the present method of choice for examining the brain.

Spine

A major advantage of MRI is that the spinal cord within the thecal sac is well-visualized without the administration of contrast media. For example, congenital lesions such as Arnold-Chiary malformation and intraspinal tumors are demonstrated without the need for myelography or intrathecal contrast media.

MRI is proving to be the gold standard in the demonstration of degenerative disk disease and lumbar disk herniation: nerve roots, neural foramina and intervertebral disk spaces are better evaluated on MRI images.

MRI of the Thorax

Because of the relatively long data acquisition time, MRI is more applicable for static parts of the body rather than for moving parts. This means that small lung lesions may be missed, but large or immobile lesions near the mediastinum are demonstrated.

Mediastinum and Hili

MRI appears to be superior to CT in the evaluation of the mediastinum and hili due to its higher contrast resolution. This can be attributed to the low signal (black) from flowing blood within the vessel providing a good intrinsic contrast to other hilar structures.

Breast, Chest Wall and Pleura

There is a remarkable similarity in the morphological appearance of MRI and mammography as both the glandular and fibrous structures are delineated by the stronger signal from surrounding fat.

Although primary tumors of the chest wall and pleura are detected with MRI, there is no superiority of this modality over CT. A disadvantage of MRI is its inability to demonstrate small calcifications.

Cardiovascular and Flow Studies

Cardiac–gated images display impressive anatomical details of the heart, as well as changes in the arterial lumen. MRI is able to depict tumors and congenital anomalies. Recent advances in MRI equipment and software, has enabled the evaluation of coronary arteries on MR angiography.

Myocardium

Acute myocardial infarction is seen as a region of high signal intensity on MR images.

Flow Studies

On flow studies, the vascular structures are defined with superb anatomical detail. The administration of contrast media is not necessary due to the intrinsic contrast between the low/black signal of flowing blood and the vascular wall. The sensitivity of the vascular tree is increased through the administration of contrast media.

However, MRI is not the final answer to all cardiac imaging as the relationship of MRI to other noninvasive imaging techniques, i.e. ultrasonography and isotope image, remains to be defined.

Abdominal MRI

The contours of organs, surrounded by fat, are well-displayed. However, the intestinal tract is not well-delineated on MRI images as bowel motion cannot be reduced through the application of a gating technique and a satisfactory oral contrast medium for the intestinal tract is not yet available.

Liver

Solid regions are detected equally well on both MRI and CT imaging. However the relationship to vascular structures is better displayed on MRI whilst the demonstration of calcified foci in tumors is better on CT than MRI. The hepatic, portal and biliary systems are well-delineated on MRI with magnetic resonance pancreatography (MRCP) a well-established procedure for the evaluation of the biliary and pancreatic tree.

Kidneys

Tumors, cysts, hydronephrosis, calculi or abscesses are successfully diagnosed with MRI. The renal cortex and medulla is differentiated assisting in the diagnosis of chronic renal failure.

Ultrasound and IVU remain the first-line standard examinations for kidney disease with CT being utilized for the diagnosis and staging of malignant renal tumors. Magnetic resonance urography (MRU) is an alternative for noninvasive imaging of the ureters.

Adrenals

The ability of MRI to detect adrenal disease is comparable to CT. Whilst CT demonstrates superior spatial resolution; MRI provides superior soft tissue contrast.

Pancreas

Recent studies have established the role of MRI in the evaluation of the pancreas. T1 and T2 weighted pulse sequences are helpful in differentiating pancreatic islet cell tumors from normal tissue.

MRI of the Pelvis

MRI of the pelvis is superior to CT due to minimal motion artefact in this region and no beam hardening effect as in CT.

Urinary Bladder

The urinary bladder is best examined when filled.

Prostatic Hypertrophy

Benign prostatic hypertrophy can be volumetrically quantified from combined multiplanar MR imaging. Prostatic cancer can be detected at an earlier stage with MRI than with CT. Endorectal coils for prostate imaging are utilized for the detection of local spread from prostatic malignancy.

The Female Pelvis

On MRI images, the uterus, ovaries and follicles are clearly displayed. The corpus uteri can be distinguished from the cervix and the myometrium is clearly differentiated from the endometrium. The changes of the endometrium in the various phases of the menstrual cycle and during pregnancy are demonstrated on MRI images.

Although MRI is currently not advocated in pregnancy, it holds great promise in the demonstration of the fetus and placental site. The ability of MRI to detect fetal metabolic disorders at an early stage has yet to be tested. The utilization of MRI for pelvimetry is possible.

The lack of known biologic hazards makes MRI an important potential tool in the management of obstetric and gynecologic problems.

Extremities and Musculoskeletal MRI

Cortical bone and epiphyseal plates appear as signal free areas, whilst normal bone marrow is seen as high signal intensity on MRI images. Conventional radiographic techniques are still superior for the demonstration of bone lesions and fractures. However fat suppressed MRI pulse sequences are highly sensitive in the detection of fractures.

The advantage of musculoskeletal examination by MRI is the superior soft tissue contrast. Fat, muscle, tendons, ligaments, nerves and blood vessels have different MRI characteristics and are separately displayed.

In joints, MRI differentiates between fluid collections of different etiologies. For example, infection, blood, serous fluid, osteomyelitis and bone marrow tumors are better characterized with MRI. Whilst the normal bone marrow gives high MRI signals, the intensity of metastatic infiltrated bone marrow is low.

Seven

Artifacts

Artifacts may be defined as the false features in the image produced during the imaging process. The random fluctuation of intensity due to noise can be considered separately from artifacts. Artifacts can be rectified easily when the causes are known. It is necessary to be familiar with specific artifacts since they can conceal pathological elements or simulate pathology that does not exists.

Artifacts can be classified into different categories, *viz.*

- Aliasing
- Chemical shift
- Gibbs/truncation
- Magic angle
- Motion
- Point
- Slice overlap
- Susceptibility
- Zipper
- Array processing
- Coil selection

Wrap Around/Aliasing

Wrap around or aliasing appears when the diameter of the scanned area is greater than the dimensions of the field of view used a part of the image is 'folded' on it self.

Fold over artifacts also known as :

i. Back folding
ii. Aliasing
iii. Wrap around artifact

Phase of the signal just out side of the field of view, increase FOV, changes preparation direction increased phase encoding.

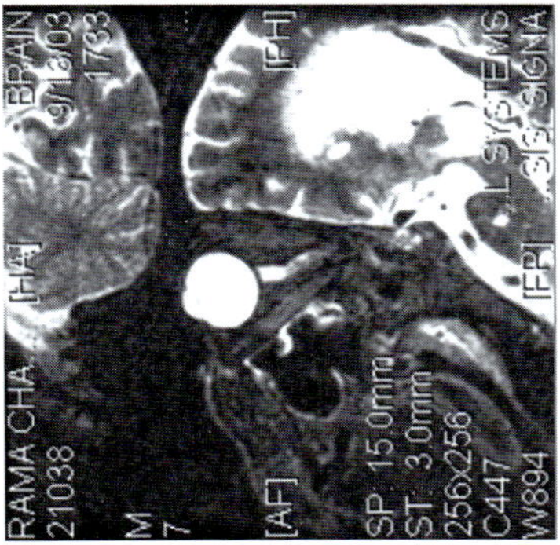

Fig. 7.1: FOV: 18 cm Aliasing of the back of the head onto the forehead in the phase direction is seen

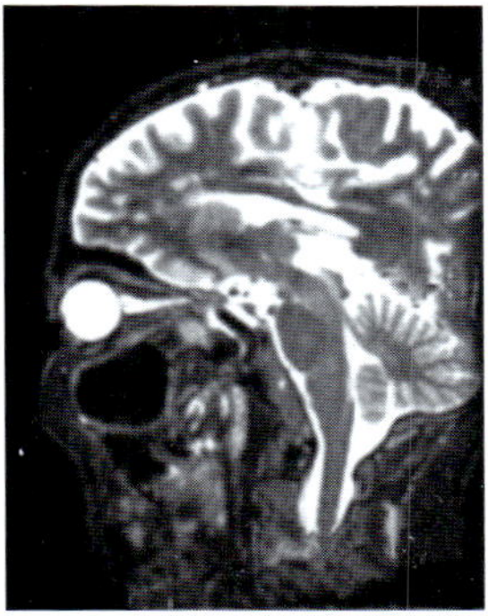

Fig. 7.2: FOV: 32 cm

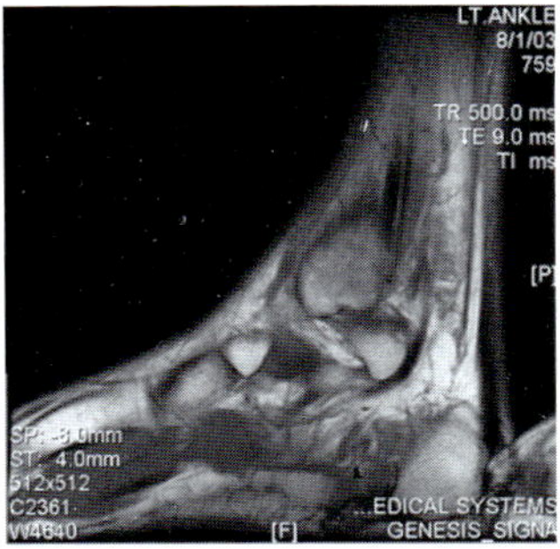

Fig. 7.3: Back folding artifact

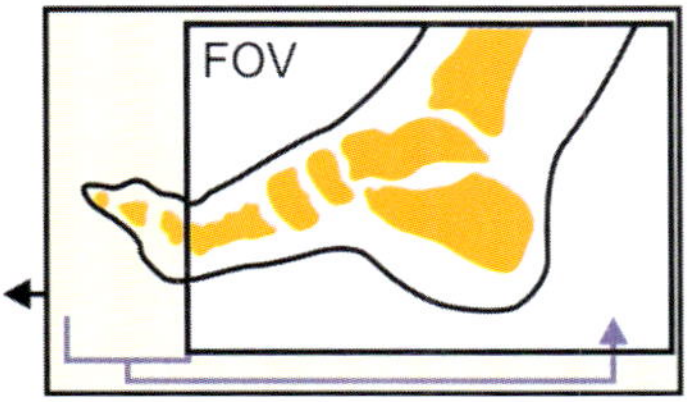

Fig. 7.4: Fold over artifact

Remedies

1. Increase FOV
2. Filtering the frequency encoded direction
3. Oversampling in the phase encoded direction

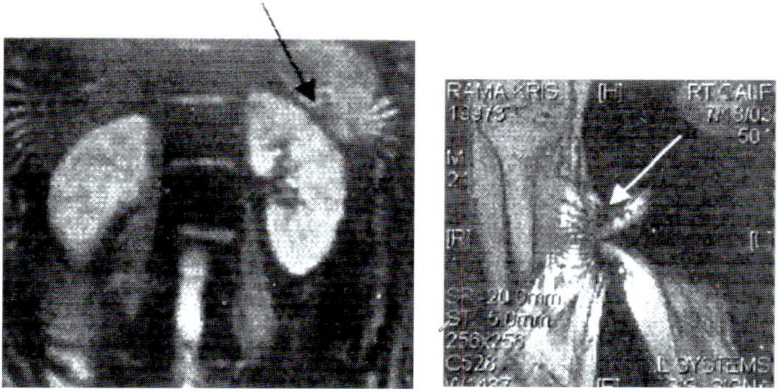

Figs 7.5A and B: Tissues outside the FOV are folded back and appear other side of the image (zebra type)

Chemical Shift Artifacts

Chemical shift artifacts appear at the interfaces between water and fat because the precessional frequency of protons is slightly different in these two substances. This leads to misregistration of the signals. They are displayed by the equipment as dark region of signal void on one side of water containing tissue and a region of bright signal at the other end of the water fat interface due to super imposition of fat and water signals on the frequency encoding direction.

The chemical shift artifacts is commonly noticed in the abdomen, spine and orbits where fat and other tissues from boarders.

This artifact is greater at higher field strengths and can be reduced by increasing the bandwidth.

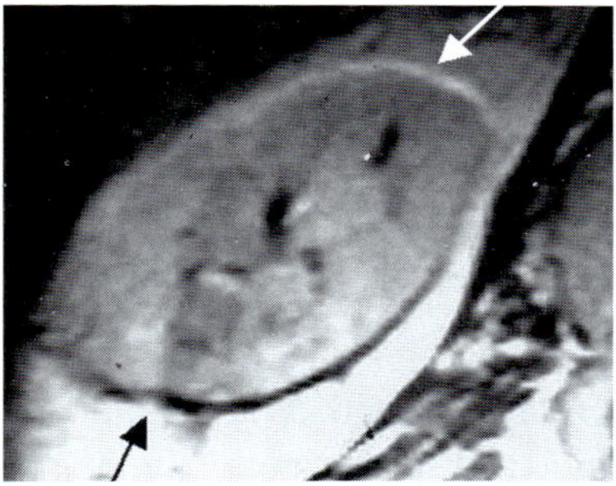

Fig. 7.6: Chemical shift misregistration artifact water in the kidneys is misregistered along the frequency axis. This causes black signal (arrow) voids at the kidneys left margins and white lines at their right margin (arrow)

The only way to eliminate this artifact is to use a fat suppression technique.

Gibbs or Truncation Artifacts

Gibbs or Truncation artifacts are bright and dark lines that are seen parallel and adjacent to boarders of abrupt intensity

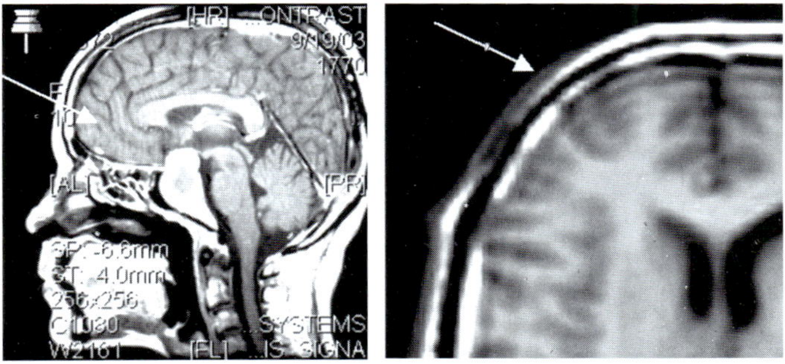

Figs 7.7A and B: Low intensity lines appearing near the boundaries of the brain/skull interface, are characteristic of a 160 phase encoding acquisition

change, as many be seen at CSF, spinal cord, fat and muscle.

These artifacts are commonly seen in phase encoding direction. They can be reduced by

a. Increasing the matrix
b. Using a filter
c. Change the direction of phase and frequency.

Magic Angle Artifacts

Magic angle artifact is seen mostly in tendons and ligaments of knee-joint that are oriented at a magic angle, i.e. 55° to the main magnetic field. This artifact is seen commonly in the rotator cuff and occasionally in the patellar tendon region and elsewhere.

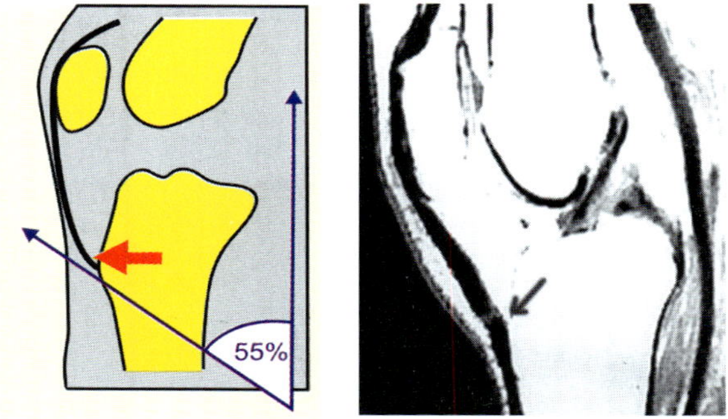

Fig. 7.8: Magic angle artifacts

Motion Artifact

Motion artifacts appear as repeating densities oriented in the phase direction occurring as the results of motion during acquisition of a sequence. These artifacts may be seen from arterial pulsations, swallowing, breathing, peristalsis and physical movement of a patient.

This type of artifact is caused by the motion of the patient voluntarily on involuntarily during the scanning. The various types of motion artifacts are as follows:

Patient motion Since all the images in one sequence are taken at the same time, it is important not to use excessively long sequences, as movement for a brief period spoils all the images.

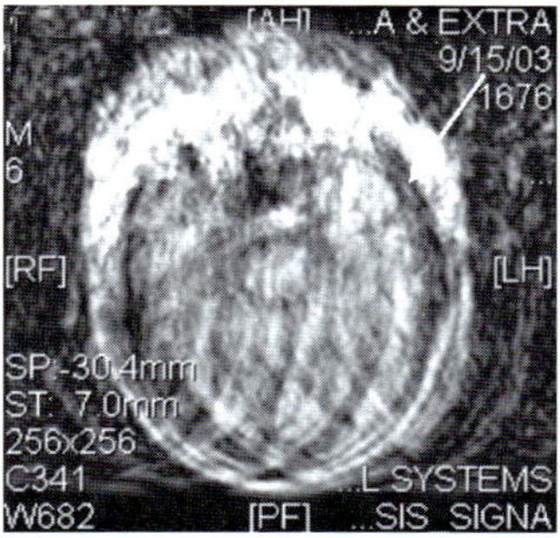

Fig. 7.9: Patient moving head. Axial section of the brain caused by motion of the head

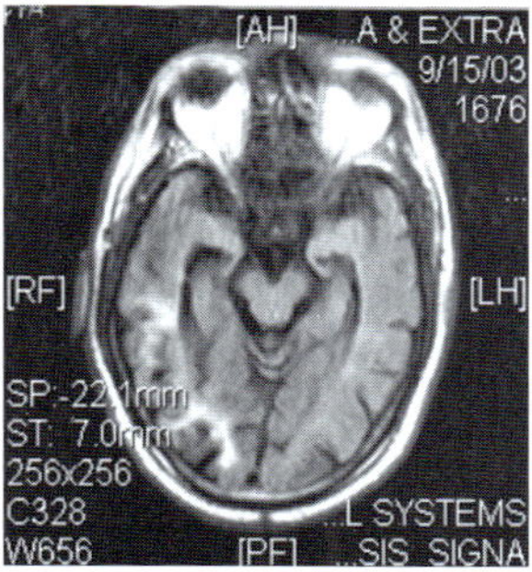

Fig. 7.10: Patient lying still

Remedy: Make patient lie comfortably, stabilize, with straps and cushions.

Cardiac motion This type of artifact is caused by the contraction and relaxation of heart (chest) while the scanning is going on.

Remedy: To avoid this type of artifact, cardiac gating is mandatory during the procedure.

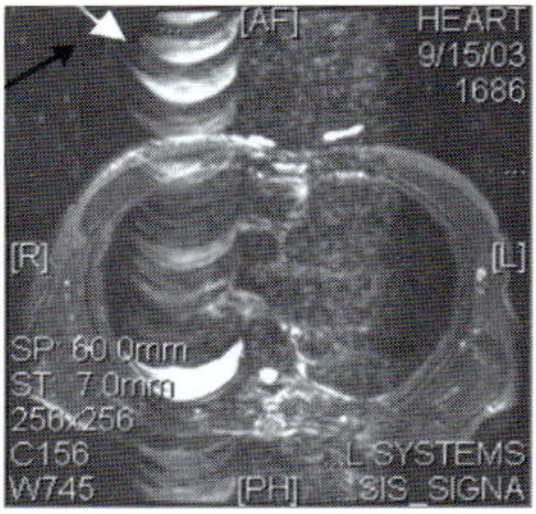

Fig. 7.11: Motion of the heart has produced ghost images without cardiac synchronization, (ECG)

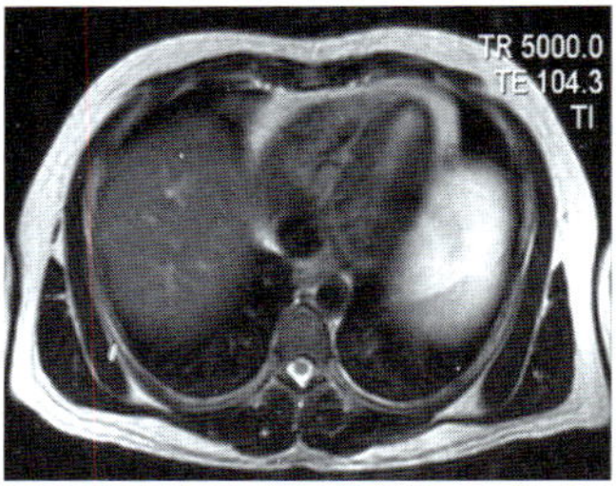

Fig. 7.12: With cardiac synchronization

Respiratory motion This type of artifact is caused by respiration during the scanning.

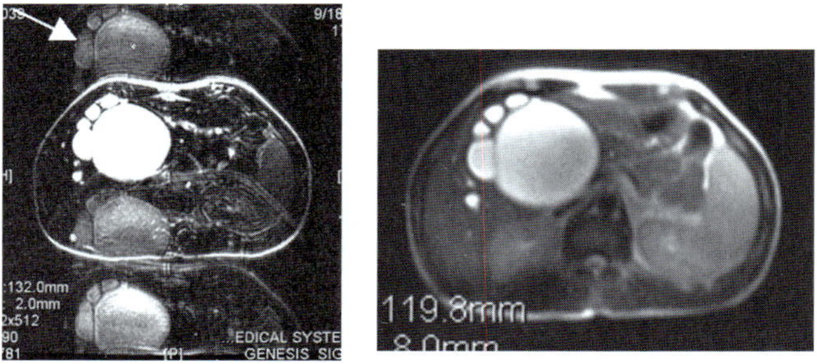

No breath hold

Breath hold

Figs 7.13A and B: Respiration-induced artifact on axial section of the abdomen. (This can be corrected by breath holding)

Remedy: This can be avoided by respiratory gating and respiratory compensation. It can be avoided by placing bellows (pressure transducers) around the patient's chest or abdomen.

Blood flow motion This type of artifact is caused by the flow of blood throughout the cardiac cycle. The artifact are prominent in axial images.

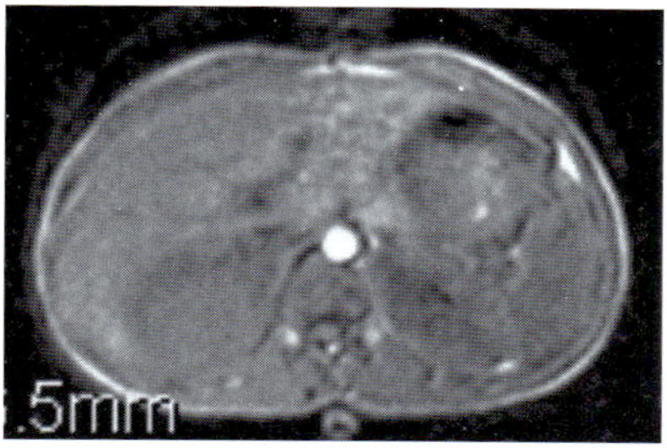

Fig. 7.14: On spoiled gradient echo images, the distance between aorta and ghost artifacts (without triggering)

Remedy: An effective remedy for blood flow motion artifact is 'Spatial Presaturation (SAT)'.

CSF pulsation The remedy for CSF pulsation ghosting is 'Gating' to the cardiac cycle, e.g. plethysmograph (peripheral gating). However, combination of 'Gating' and flow compensation (flow comp) is optimal for cervical and thoracic imaging.

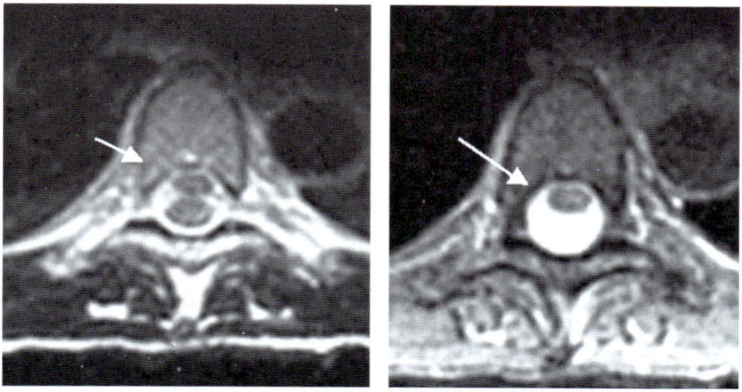

Figs 7.15A and B: Transversal image of the T spine showing flow voids in CSF

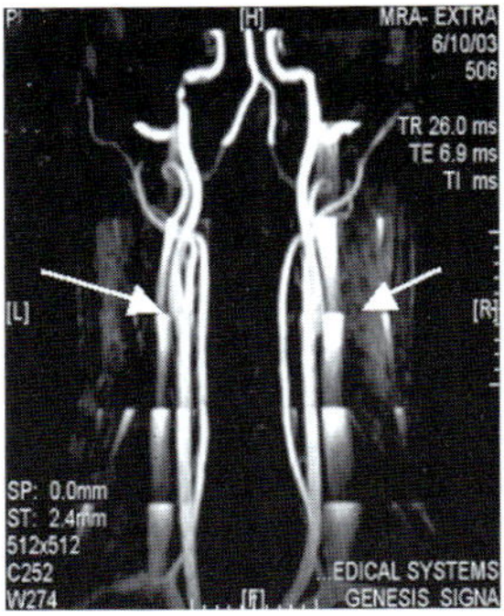

Fig. 7.16: Image showing step artifact due to MOTSA (3D TOF)

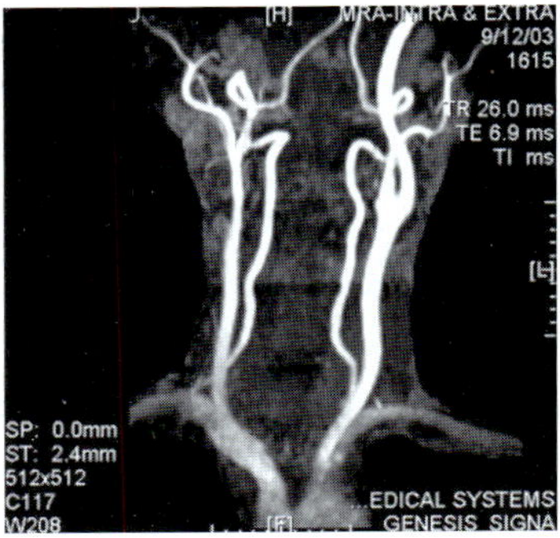

Fig. 7.17: Postcontrast smart prep.

3D TOF MOTSA Three dimensional TOF and multiple overlapping thin slab acquisitions (MOTSA) images of the neck. Patient motion and vascular pulsations during acquisition resulted in a stair-step pattern in the 3D TOF of MIP. The MOTSA images have higher SNR but greater background signal.

Aperiodic motion This type of artifact is caused by the involuntary motion of the patient like peristalsis, swallowing and blinking of the eye.

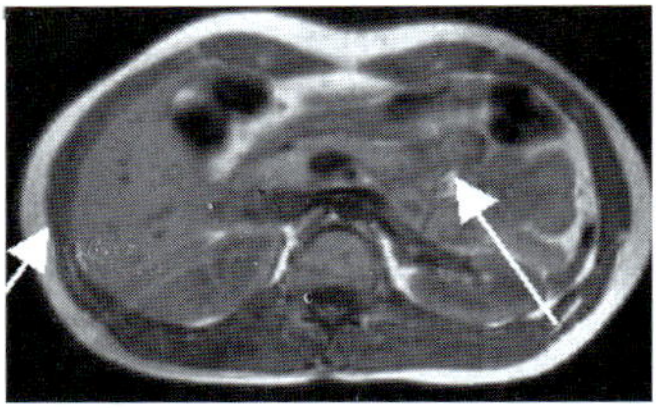

Fig. 7.18: Without respiratory compensation

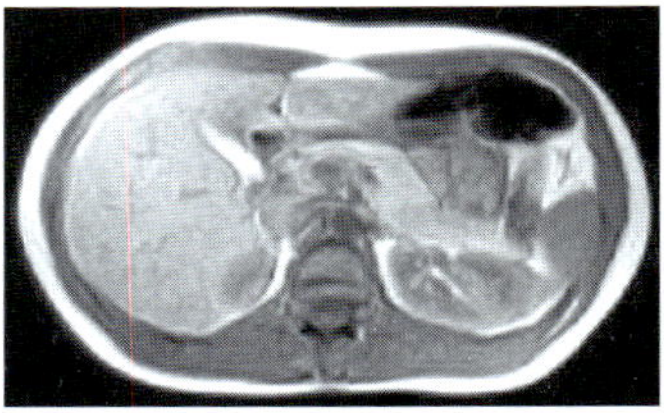

Fig. 7.19: With respiratory compensation

Arrow shows motion of the abdomen has produced several curved lines

Remedy: Except for peristalsis, the patient motion is best controlled by cooperation and suitable education.

In order to reduce the motion artifacts caused by bowel movement administration of Glucagon (IV) or Buscopan (IM). Preprocedural is advisable.

Point Artifact

Point artifact is seen as a bright spot of increased signal intensity in the center of the image. This is caused due to constant offset of DC voltage in the receiver coil which after Fourier transformation appear as a bright spot in the center of the image.

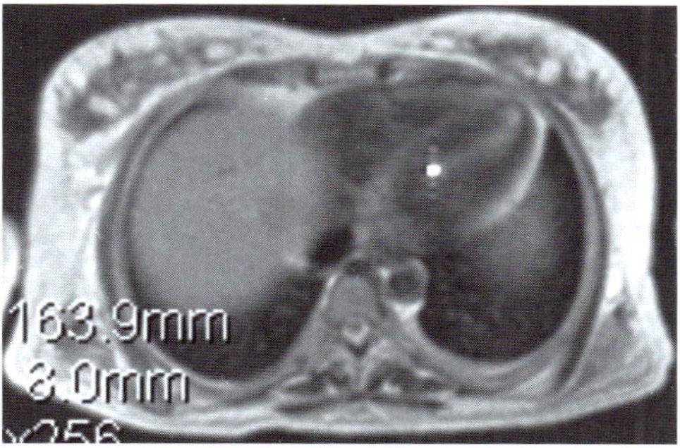

Fig. 7.20: This is an axial image of the cardiac showing a central point artifact

Slice Overlap Artifact

The slice overlap artifact is a name given to the loss of signal seen in an image from a multiangle, multislice acquisitions, as is obtained commonly in the lumbar spine.

If the slices obtained at different disk spaces are not parallel, then the slices may overlap.

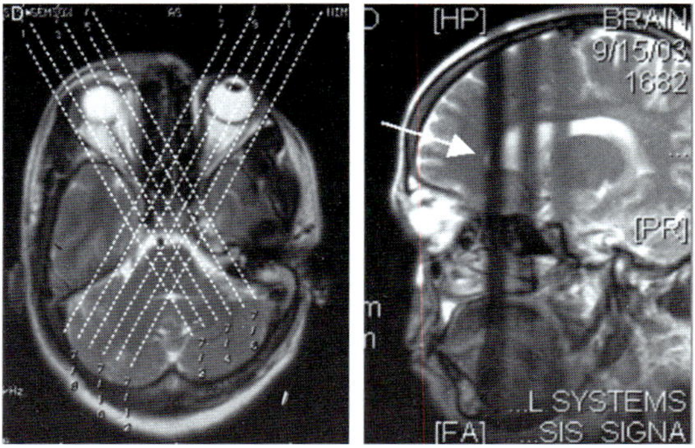

Figs 7.21A and B: Para-axials (oblique) T2 weighted images through optic nerves from a multiangle. This causes a band of signal loss crossing vertically in sagittal image

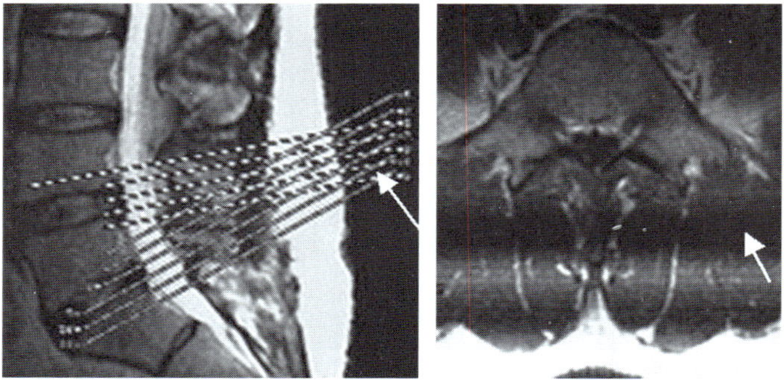

Arrow shows signal loss from overlap

Figs 7.22A and B: This is a para-axial T2 weighted image through L5/S1 from a multiangle, multislice acquisition, as is obtained commonly in the lumbar spine

If two levels are done at the same time, e.g. L4/L5 and L5/S1 then the level acquired second will include spins that have already been saturated. This causes a band of signal loss crossing horizontally or vertically in our image, usually prominent posteriorly.

Susceptibility Artifacts

The susceptibility of a tissue fells us how easily it can be magnetized. Normally most of the tissues have susceptibility values which fall in a fairly narrow range. However, presence of paramagnetic material like hemoglobin degradation products or tissue-air interphases lead to local

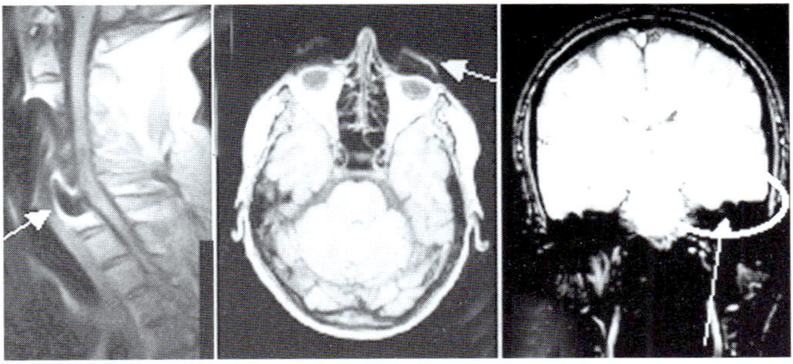

A Make up eyeliner

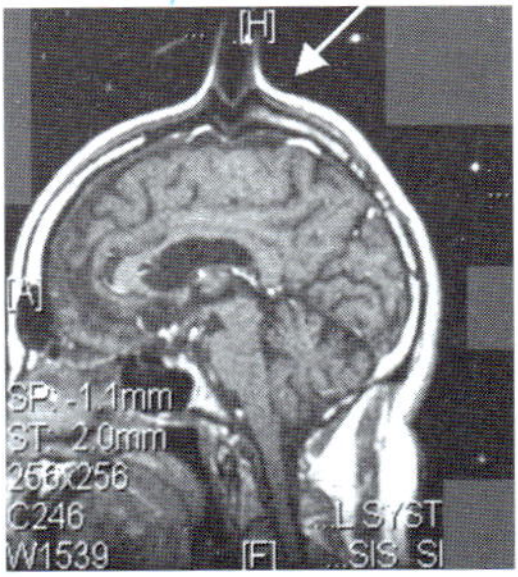

B Magnetic field distortion due to hair pin

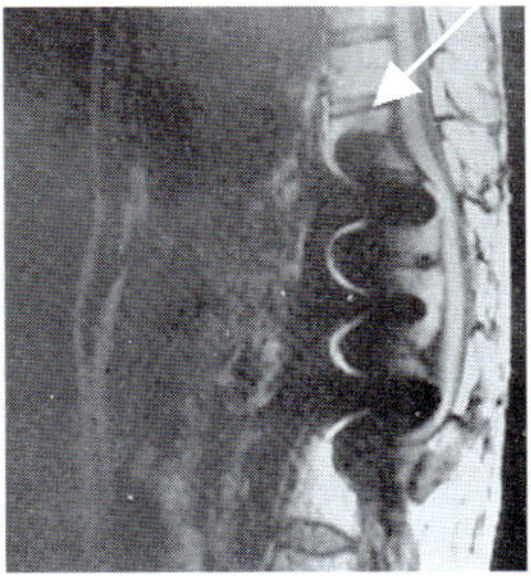

C Harrington rod

Figs 7.23A to C: Arrows indicate distortion due to susceptibility differences between metal and body tissue. Artifacts caused by metallic objects, causing severe signal loss and geometric distortion

variations in the susceptibility. This is turn results in reduction in the quality of the local field.

Tissue air interphases related artifacts are commonly seen around the para nasal sinuses and the lungs. These susceptibility artifacts can be removed by using spin echo-sequences.

Zipper Artifacts

This artifact is caused by external RF entering the room at a certain frequency and interfering with inherently weak signal coming from the patient.

There are various causes for zipper artifacts in images. Most of them are related to hardware or software problems. The zipper artifacts that can be controlled easily are those due to RF entering the scanning room when the door is open during acquisition of images.

RF from radio transmitters will cause zipper artifacts that are oriented perpendicular to the frequency axis of the image.

Frequently there is more than one artifact line on an image from this cause.

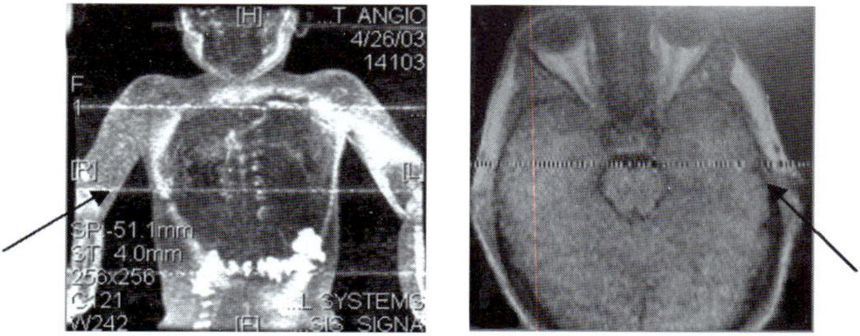

Figs 7.24A and B: Effect of right interface causing streak artifacts. This can be caused by a leaking RF, causing pick-up of external RF signals

Remedy: System generated artifacts should be reported service engineer.

IMPROPER COIL SELECTION

Select a proper suitable coil, if you do not enter correct one, the system will create noise on image. Structured noise caused due to coil selection.

Select a coil from the coil name window.

The coil selected should match the one that is connected.

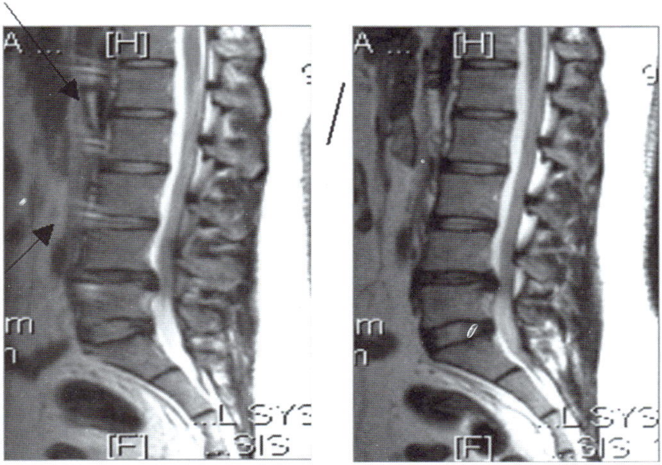

Arrows show artifact (Improper selection of coil)
A. CTL — Bottom coil

Without artifact (Proper selection of coil)
B. CTL — 456 coil

Figs 7.25A and B: An example of lumbar spine sagittal image is shown in Fig (a)

Array Processing Artifact

The array processor (AP) is part of the computation system. It is a very fast parallel processor for execution of simultaneous tasks. The array processor is involved in the signal averaging process during data acquisition and reconstruction.

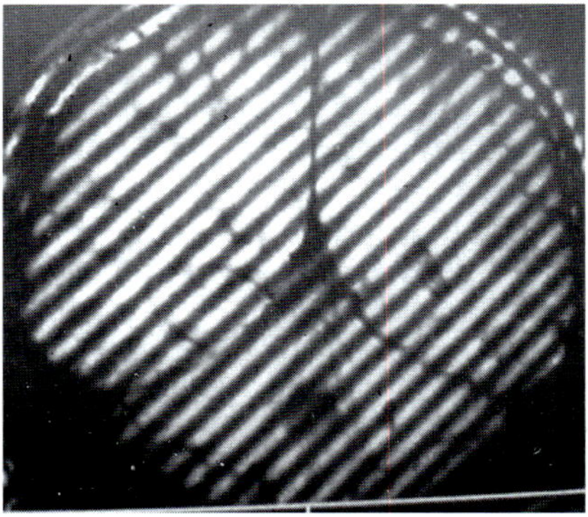

Fig. 7.26: Coronal T2 weighted spin echo image of the head. Grid-like artifacts superimposed on the image are characteristic of a faulty array processor

Eight

Technical Factors Influencing the Image Quality

INTRODUCTION

There are many factors available to the technologist when setting up a sequence. The appropriate selection of the parameters determines the weighting, improved quality of images and sensitivity to pathology. Therefore, the technologist should be aware of these factors and their interrelation so that optimal quality of the images can be obtained. The following are the factors discussed below which affect the quality of the image.

Performing an MR examination demands multiple choices:

i. The acquisition parameters
ii. The imaging plane orientation,
   Type of coil, slice thickness, matrix size, number of excitations, etc.

FACTORS AFFECTING THE SNR

Field of View (FOV)

FOV is one of the important factors affecting the SNR.

An image consists of a FOV that relates to the region of interest (anatomy) covered.

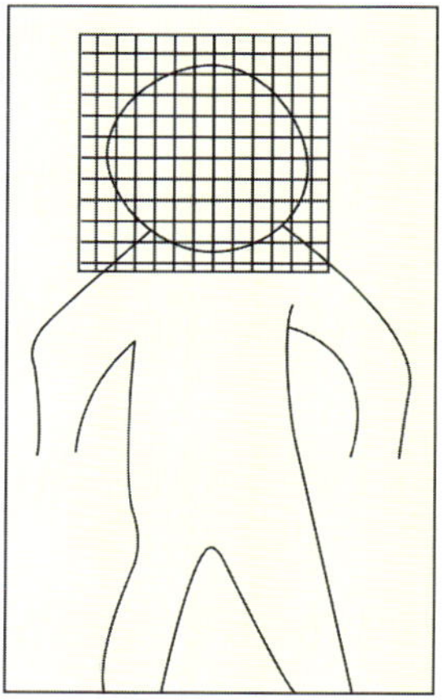

Fig. 8.1: Field of view (FOV)

The field of view ranges from 10 to 50 cm for most of the equipment. Therefore, if the entire spinal cord is to be imaged in the sagittal plane, its upper and lower parts need complementary series of pulse sequences.

FOV controls spatial resolution and SNR.

Small FOV produces ↑ (high) resolution ↓ (low) SNR and increases the minimum TE value = SAT pulses decreases the number of slices in an acquisition.

At a given matrix size (i.e. number of pixels on the two image coordinates), the FOV determines pixel size, e.g. at a FOV of 24 cm and a matrix size of 256 × 256 pixels, the pixel size is 0.9 mm × 0.9 mm (240 mm/256).

FOV = 175 mm	FOV = 325 mm
High resolution	Low resolution
SNR = 100 percent	SNR = 345 percent

It is critical that the technologist should understand the relationship between signal-to-noise and FOV. SNR is proportional to square of the FOV.

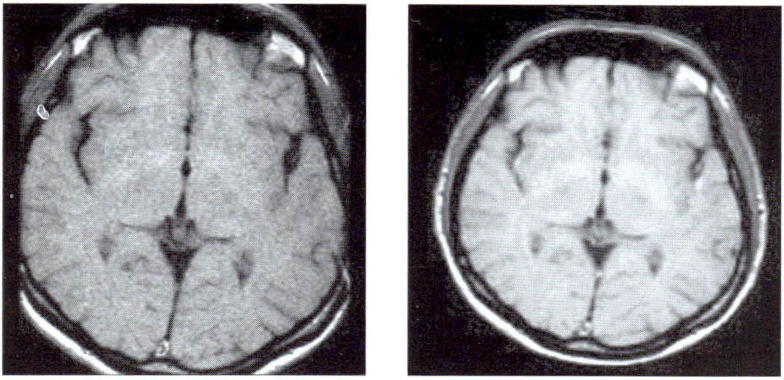

FOV: 12 cm FOV: 24 cm

Figs 8.2A and B: SNR ~ FOV^2

For example, Having a FOV reduced from 24 to 12 cm results in, a signal-to-noise reduction of 75 percent.

In practice, the reduction in FOV requires some change that results in increased SNR.

Spatial Resolution

Spatial resolution is defined as the ability to separate closely spaced anatomical details.

Slice Thickness

To give each slice a thickness, a band of nuclei must be excited by the excitation pulse.

Increase of slice thickness, increases SNR, coverage of anatomy and partial volume whereas spatial resolution is decreased.

As slice thickness ↑ (increases), resolution ↓ (decreases) and SNR ↑ (increases).

Decrease of slice thickness, reduces SNR, coverage of anatomy and partial volume whereas spatial resolution is increased.

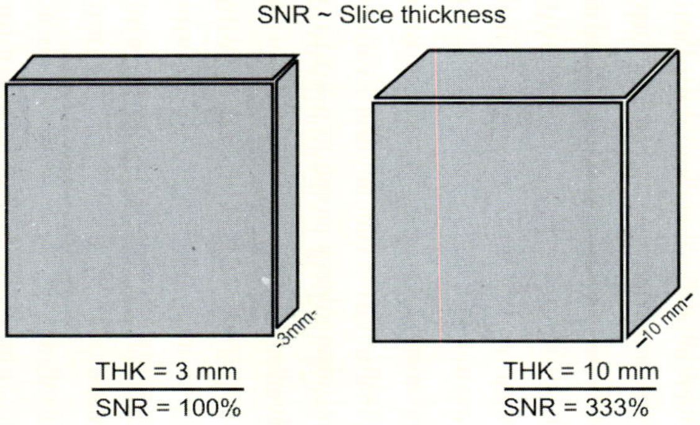

Figs 8.3A and B: SNR ~ slice thickness

The basic values of slice thickness ranges from 3 to 15 mm.

Slice thickness controls resolution and SNR.

The technologist should be aware that as the slice thickness is increased or decreased, there will be a corresponding change in the S/N ratio for the image.

If one slice is acquired at a 6 mm thickness, and another slice is acquired at a 3 mm thickness (with all other factors equal), the second slice will have one-half the signal of the first slice. Since the noise is essentially unchanged, the effect is that the S/N ratio will be cut in half for the second slice.

SNR ~ SLICE THICKNESS

Thickness = 3 mm	Thickness = 10 mm
SNR = 50 percent	SNR = 167 percent
Scan time = 1.28 sec	Scan time = 1.28 sec

Ideally, we would like to obtain images from, infinitely thin sections. The thicker the slice, the more partial volume,

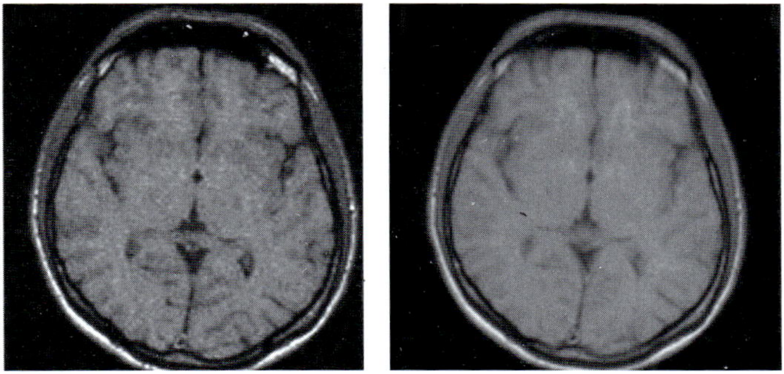

Figs 8.4A and B: SNR ~ slice thickness

which implies that certain structures may be hidden by overlying tissues.

On the other hand, SNR and CNR are improved for larger slice thickness.

Spacing

Spacing is the gap between two slices. When acquiring a multiplanar, single acquisition, spacing controls cross-talk.

As spacing ↑ (increases), cross-talk ↓ (decreases)

Typically, a spacing that is 20 percent of the slice thickness is sufficient to minimize cross-talk.

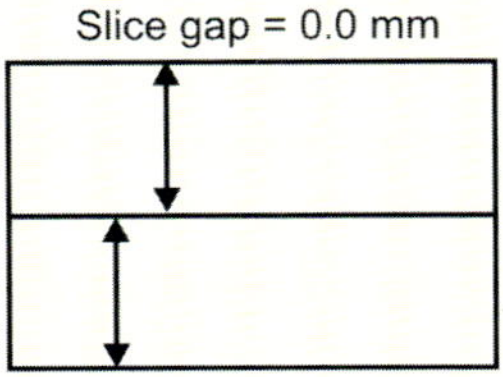

Fig. 8.5A: Contiguous slices

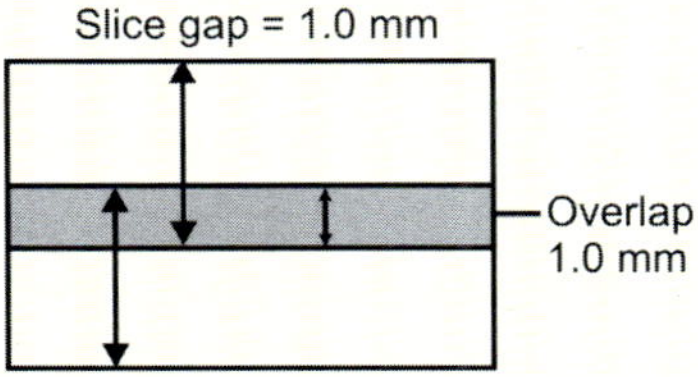

Fig. 8.5B: Overlapping slices

As no.of slices ↑ (increases), scan time also ↑ (increases)

Ideally, we would like to obtain our images from completely contiguous slices. In practice, there is always some excitation outside the slice boundaries. This means that when exciting a particular slice with a RF pulse, partial excitation of neighboring slices will cause an alteration in image contrast, or the effective TR for every slice is less than determined by TR.

Matrix Size

The matrix size is represented by two figures. The first figure usually relates to the number of frequency samples taken, whereas the second relates to the number of phase encodings performed. For example 256 × 128 indicates that 256 frequency samples are taken during readout and 128 phase encodings are performed. A course matrix corresponds to less number of pixels and fine matrix corresponds to more number of pixels.

In all digital imaging methods, and therefore in MR too, the image is divided into small picture elements called pixels. Each individual pixel corresponds to the intensity and amplitude of MR signal represented on gray scale.

The dimensions of the matrix can be changed. The most commonly used matrix is 256 × 256. Some systems offer low-resolution (128 × 128) and or/high-resolution (512 × 512) matrixes.

At a given FOV, matrix size determines pixel size and thus spatial resolution.

Therefore, an image obtained with 128 × 256 pixels is typically less well resolved in the Y dimension than one obtained with 256 × 256 pixels. However, all other para-

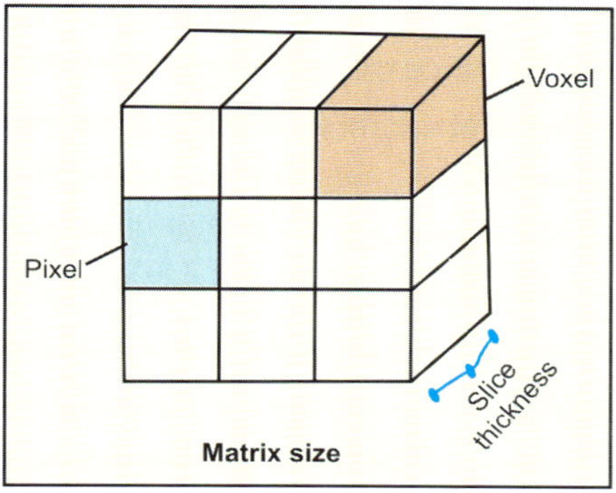

Fig. 8.6

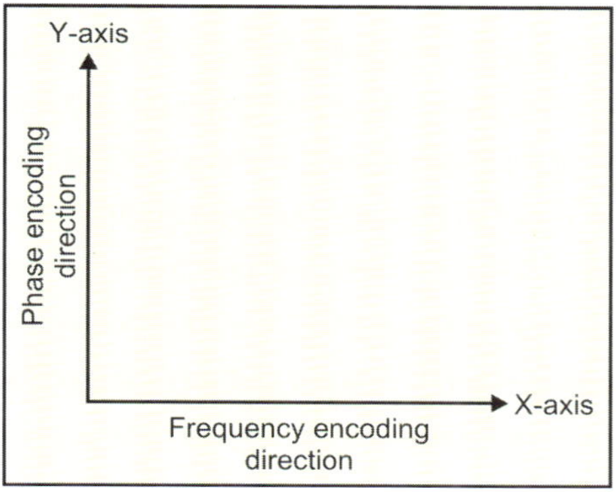

Fig. 8.7

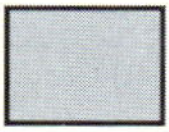

$$\text{Pixel size} = \frac{\text{Field of view (FOV)}}{\text{Matrix size (MS)}}$$

Fig. 8.8

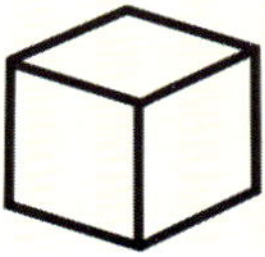

$$\text{Voxel size} = \text{Thickness} \times \frac{\text{FOV}^2}{\text{MS}^2}$$

Fig. 8.9

meters being equal, the 256 × 256 image has a factor of 2 less SNR, while it requires twice the scan time.

Pixel: Acronym for a picture element, the smallest discrete part of a digital image display.

Voxel: Volume element, the element of the three-dimensional space (3D-space) corresponding to a pixel, for a given slice thickness.

Scan Time ~ Matrix Size

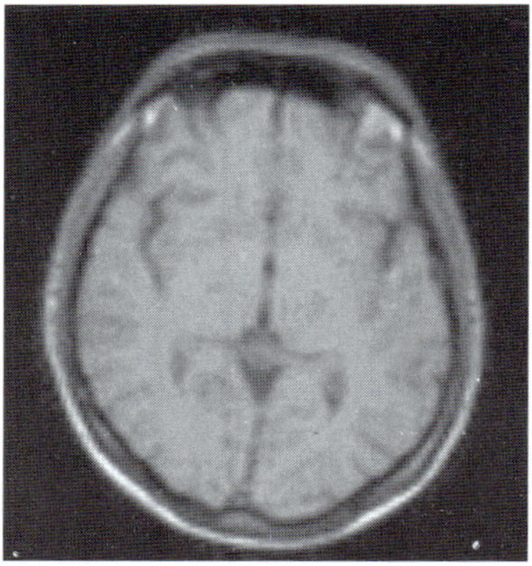

Fig. 8.10

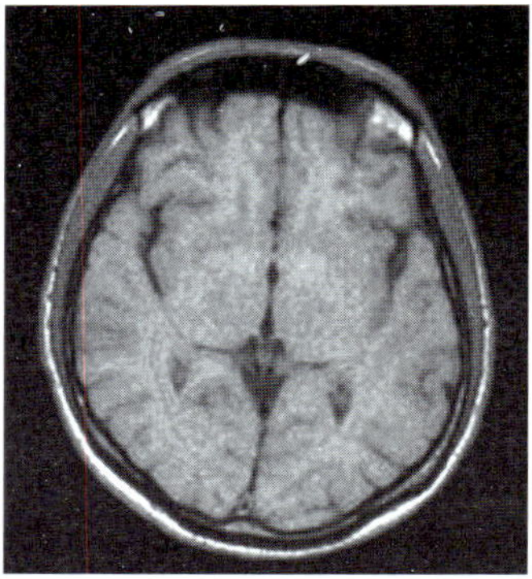

Fig. 8.11

Scan time ~ matrix size

Matrix size = 256 mm
Good resolution
SNR = 100 percent
Time: 2 min

Matrix size = 512 mm
High resolution
SNR = 25 percent
Time: 4 min

Prescan

Prescanning is a method of calibration to be performed prior to every data acquisition. The following are the three main tasks involved in prescanning *viz.*

i. Finding out the center frequency at which RF is to be transmitted.
ii. Finding the exact magnitude of radiofrequency ought to be transmitted in order to generate maximum signal in the coil.
iii. Adjustment of the magnitude of the received signal.

Prescan allows for the adjustment of the transmit and receive gain and the setting of the center frequency for a specific body part to be imaged.

Number of Excitations or Number of Signal Averages (NEX/NSA)

Every individual signal which contributes to form a MR image, can be received once or collected several times using repeated excitations. Hence, the average signal value is used to generate the image. When the number of excitations are increased, the error (the noise) doubt and the measurements are more precise.

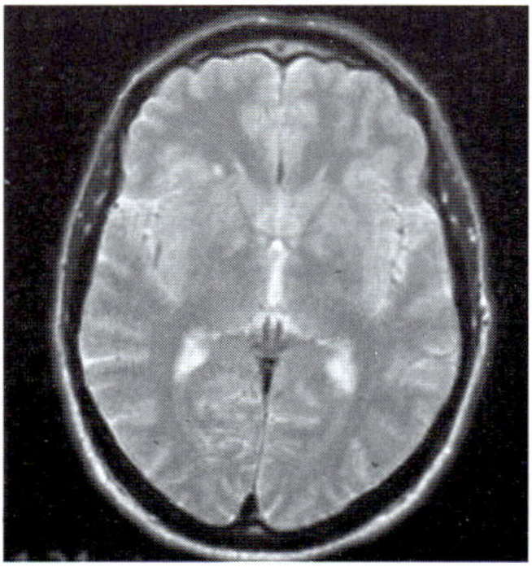

Fig. 8.12

Nex = 2
Scan time = 1.28 min
SNR = 100 percent

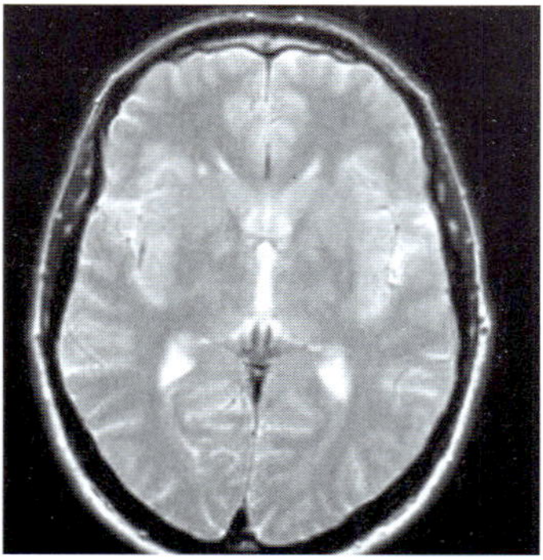

Fig. 8.13

Nex = 4
Scan time = 2.48 min
SNR = 141 percent

In practice, the number of excitations ranges from 1 to 6.

The number of excitations (Nex) implies the number of times a particular line in sampled in K space. K space refers to the raw data of an image.

A line in K space corresponds to the spin echo obtained at a particular setting of the phase encoding gradient. Scan time is proportional to Nex.

By increasing the number of excitations, the SNR is improved and *vice versa*.

Image Acquisition Time (Examination Time)

The longer the scan time, the more chances that the patient moves and generates, more artifacts that prevent the interpretation of the images. Hence, optimum scanning time is to be maintained so that appreciable quality of images can be obtained which are free of artifacts (motion artifacts).

For a given patient, the duration of an MR examination depends on several factors.

- Getting the patient settled and centering the area to be studied.
- The number of areas to be examined.
- The number and characteristics of the pulse sequences used.
- The acquisition time (T) of a sequence is given by the following formula:

$$\boxed{\text{Acquisition Time (T)} = \text{TR} \times \text{N} \times \text{Nex}}$$

Where, TR is the repetition time,
N is the number of phase encodings in the matrix
Nex is the number of excitations

$$\begin{aligned}\text{Acquisition Time} &= \text{TR} \times \text{N} \times \text{Nex}\\ &= 400 \times 160 \times 2\end{aligned}$$

= 128 sec
= 2.14 minutes

Image (Data) Acquisition Time

The time required to gather a complete set of image data. The total time for performing a scan must be taken into consideration. The additional image reconstruction time when determining how quickly the image(s) may be viewed.

Increase of TR increases the scan time and similarly increasing the number of phase encodings in a matrix increases the scan time and *vice versa*.

Improving the SNR by increasing Nex also increases the imaging time and *vice versa*.

Frequency

Frequency axis of the acquisiton matrix.

The number of cycles or separations of a periodic process per unit time. In electromagnetic radiation, it is usually expressed in units of Hertz (Hz), where 1 Hz = 1 cycle.

Increase the frequency matrix to produce (high) resolution, ↓ (low) SNR and ↓ less number of slices.

Phase

In a periodic function (such as rotational or sinusoidal motion), the position relative to a particular part of the cycle.

Phase controls scan time for most pulse sequence data base and may control resolution.

Nex: Select a Nex value that produces sufficient SNR.

Phase FOV

PFOV shortens scan time by scaling down the FOV size in the phase direction.

Select 0.75 or 0.5 to reduce phase steps and thus

↓ (less) Scan time
↓ (less) FOV in the Phase direction
↓ (decreases) SNR slightly.

Freq DIR: S/I (superior to inferior), A/P (anterior to posterior), R/L (right to left).

The scanning direction associated with the frequency gradient.

The direction displayed is the default frequency direction which is typically the long axis of the image.

To swap phase and frequency, select the other direction.

Auto Shim

Auto shim is typically selected when the FOV center is not at isocenter.

A preparation phase is performed in which small gradient amplitudes are determined which optimize the main magnetic field homogeneity. The small gradients remain present during the scan.

Contrast

Select only contrast if contrast is injected. Enter amount of contrast injected and the type of contrast used in the designated fields.

Phase Correction

A process that mathematically corrects for phase errors in FSE and (EP) sequences. Phase correction is selected for EPI and FSE, FSE-IR and FLAIR protocols.

1. Corrective processing of the spectrum so that spectral lines at different frequencies all have the decorption—mode phase.
2. In imaging, adjustment of the signal in different parts of the image to have a consistent phase.

Auto Center Frequency

Select the CF peak that should be set during prescan.

A prescan procedure to fine-tune the system's RF transmit/receive frequency to the precessional frequency of the protons under study, providing optimal sampling of a patient's anatomy.

Unlike other imaging modalities, magnetic resonance (MR) imaging requires a multitude of operating parameter decisions. Improper choices can result in impaired image quality, cause artifacts and reduce a study's diagnostic efficacy. Therefore, it is important that the technologist should understand both intrinsic tissue parameters, extrinsic equipment parameters as well as how they interact.

Noise is always superimposed on the images. This noise causes a fluctuation of pixel values.

Signal-to-Noise Ratio (SNR)

It is defined as the ratio of the amplitude of the signal generated to the average amplitude of the noise. Quality of image is mainly characterized by its SNR. Increase of signal increases the SNR and *vice versa*. The following are the factors that affect the SNR:

- Coil type
- Volume of the voxel

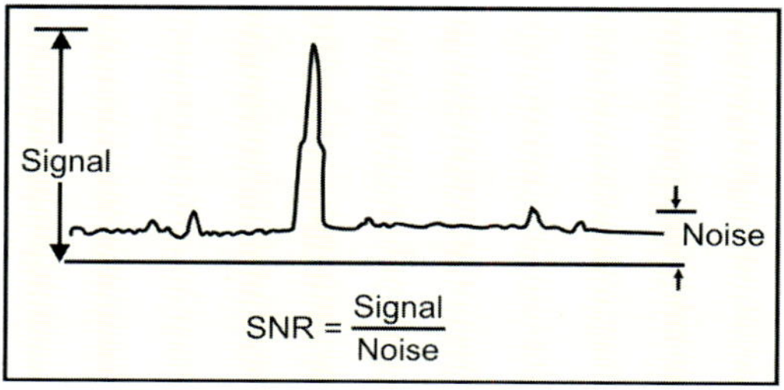

	As TR↑	As TE↑	As Nex↑	Slice thick↑	Spac-ing↑	FOV↑	Re-ceive band width↑	Phase matrix↑	Freq. matrix↑
SNR	↑	↓	↑	↑	↑	↑	↓	↑	↓

Fig. 8.14: Various factors which contributes to change of SNR

- Proton density of the region of interest under examination
- TR, TE and Flip angle
- Nex
- Receive bandwidth
- FOV

Scan time, spatial resolution, SNR are mathematically related.

Contrast-to-Noise Ratio (CNR)

It is defined as the difference in the SNR of two adjacent areas. The factors that affect CNR are the same as that of SNR.

Bandwidth (BW)

A general term referring to a range of frequencies (e.g. contained in a signal or passed by a signal processing system).

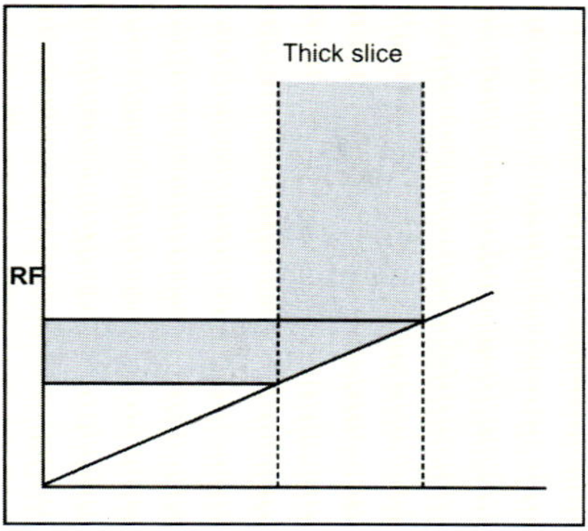

A. Large bandwidth

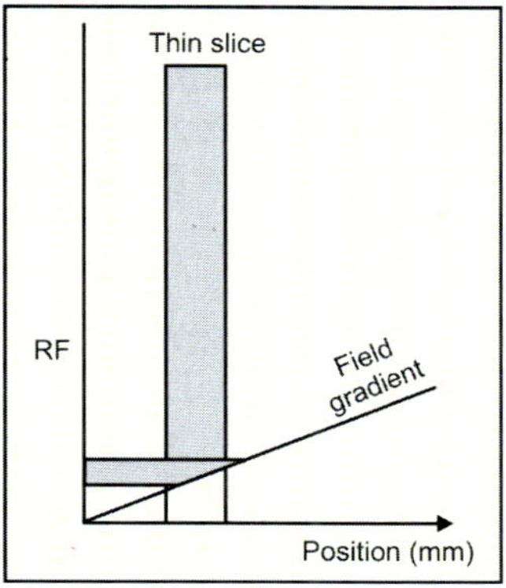

B. Small bandwidth

Figs 8.15A and B: Selecting slice thickness

This is the range of frequencies that are acquired by the readout gradient. As bandwidth is decreased, noise is reduced thereby increasing the SNR. If the bandwidth is reduced to half, SNR is increased by 40 percent but increases the sampling time.

Bandwidth defines the number of frequencies. We can change the bandwidth with RF pulses.

Frequency can be swapped with phase direction by champing the entry in (Freq DIR), following the table sum.

The default directions of phase freq. and slice select by coil selection.

Two-Dimensional Fourier Transform (2DFT)

In order to reconstruct the image, each gradient cycle (slice-selection, phase-encoding, readout) must be repeated for each level of the phase-encoding axis. For example, a matrix of 256 × 256 would require 256 cycles. Each of the 256 resulting signals (k-space data) is then converted from its time domain into its frequency domain by a Fourier Transform. Each signal produced along the horizontal axis is the sum of all the magnetization vectors for that level of the phase encoding gradient. After all 256 signals have been transformed into their frequency domain (shown below), a Fourier Transform is performed at each frequency utilizing the data at all phase encoding levels to decode the spatial information along the vertical axis. The second Fourier Transform is performed on each corresponding point along x and y, where y = the sum of all 256 signals collected at each level of the y-axis.

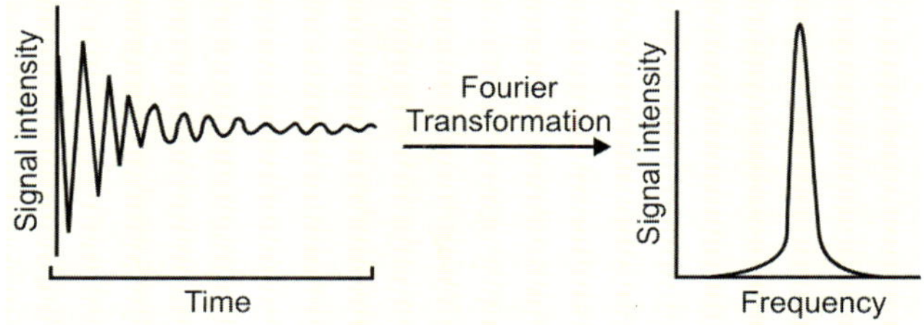

Figs 8.16A and B: Fourier transformation

Table 8.1: The default directions for phase, frequency, and slice, select by coil selection

Coil	*Plane*	*Frequency*	*Phase*	*Slice Select*
Head coil	Axial	A/P	R/L	S/I
	Sagittal	S/I	A/P	R/L
	Coronal	S/I	R/L	A/P
Body,	Axial	R/L	A/P	S/I
extremity, NV	Sagittal	S/I	A/P	R/L
Array coil,	Coronal	S/I	R/L	A/P
Surface coil				
Receive only				

Frequency can be swapped with phase direction by changing the entry in (Frequency Direction).

Image Reconstruction

The mathematical process of converting the composite signals obtained during the data acquisition phase into an image.

GRADIENTS

In order to spatially encode the NMR signal, a gradient magnetic field is superimposed on the static magnetic field. The gradients place the nuclei in a slightly different magnetic field depending on their location.

SLICE-SELECT

In order to confine excitation to a single slice only, an RF pulse containing a narrow band of frequencies is applied, in conjunction with the gradient located in the plane perpendicular to the imaging plane. In an axial image in the x-y plane, for example, the slice-selection gradient is Gz. The gradient is applied only during the RF excitation pulse. Only that plane of nuclei located with its z position such that its Larmor Frequency matches that of the applied RF will be excited to produce a signal.

Slice Orientation

Superior⟷Inferior (axial plane)
Right⟷Left (sagittal plane)
Anterior⟷Posterior (coronal plane).

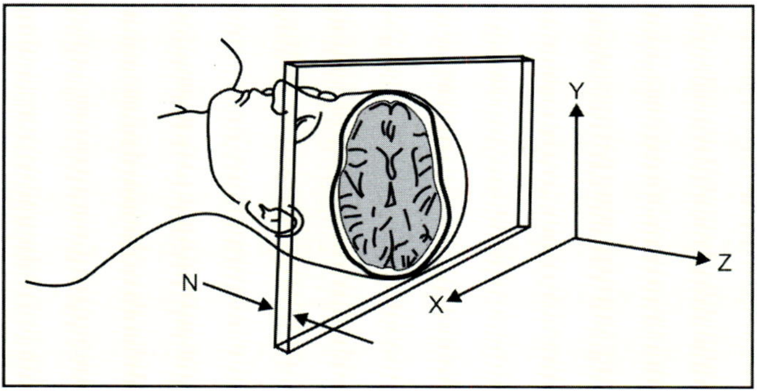

Fig. 8.17: A gradient is applied along the z-axis in conjunction with a narrow band RF pulse to confine excitation to a single slice only

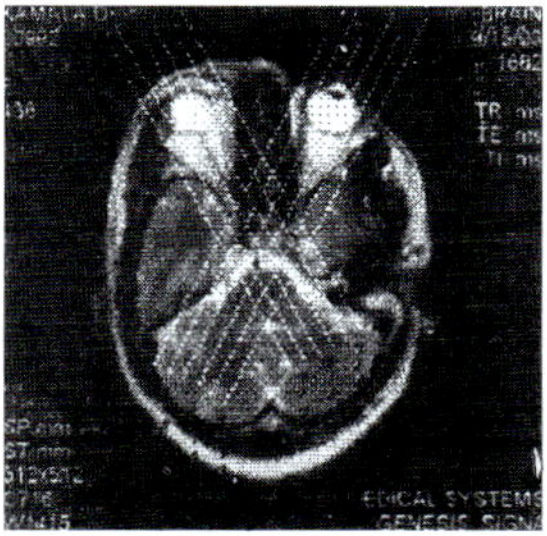

Fig. 8.18A: The orientation of simple oblique slices can be specified by rotating a slice

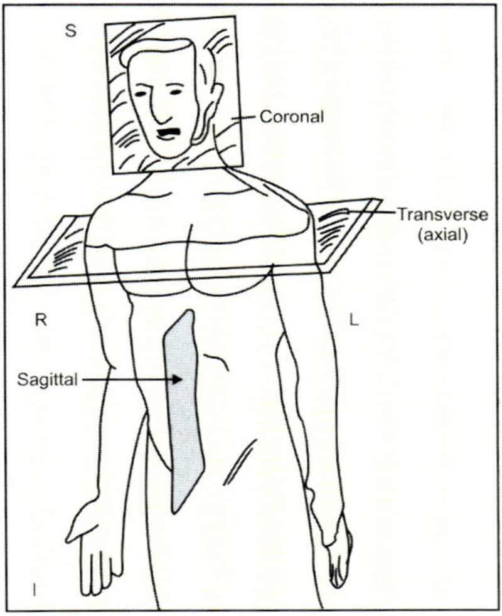

Fig. 8.18B: A plan of planes. The diagram shows the slice plane in the patient transverse, sagittal and coronal

Nine

MRI Contrast Agents

CONTRAST AGENTS

MRI provides excellent soft tissue contrast. However, enhancement with contrast agents substantially improves the sensitivity and specificity of lesions. Contrast agents are pharmaceuticals that enhance the contrast between the lesions and normal structures. Enhancement of the image contrast between normal and diseased tissue increases the diagnostic accuracy. Contrast agents are commonly used in clinical practice for a broad range of indications.

IDEAL CONTRAST

The ideal contrast agent should have the following properties:

1. The contrast agent must be efficient at low concentrations
2. The contrast agent should possesses tissue specificity to enable higher concentration in specific tissue
3. The contrast agent must be substantially chased from the targeted tissue.
4. It must have low viscosity
5. The contrast agent must possesses a suitable shelf life for storage purposes
6. It should be nontoxic.

There is no ideal contrast to date. However there are many MR contrast agents that are safe, highly effective and widely used in routine clinical practice.

HISTORY

Nearly all MR contrast agents constitute paramagnetic compounds. The most commonly used paramagnetic ion is the gadolinium (Gd) ion. This ion attaches with various ligands (chemical compounds) such as diethylenetriamine penta acetic acid (DTPA) that act as chelating agents. The reaction of Gd ions with DTPA forms a stable chelate complex. The presence of unpaired electrons in the paramagnetic ion is a mandatory component to affect changes in the T1 and T2 relaxation times of protons. The utilization of a paramagnetic ion with highest spin quantum number is desirable. The Gd ion of the lanthanide metal group has a high spin quantum number (7/2), making this ion a desirable contrast agent.

The first and foremost MRI contrast agent on the world market was Schering Magnevist, the dimeglumine salt of gadolinium–diethylenetriamine penta acetic acid (Gd-DTPA).

Presently three gadolinium based contrast agents are approved by the US Food and Drug Administration (FDA). These are nonionic Gd-DTPA-BMA (Gadodiamide or omniscan), ionic Gd-DTPA(gadopentetate dimeglumine or magnevist) and nonionic Gd-HP-DO3A (gadoteridol or prohance). The osmolarity and viscosity of each of these three contrast agents are given in Table 9.1.

Mechanism of Action

MR contrast agents alter tissue contrast. Signal will increase when hydrogen proton increases, T1 decreases

Table 9.1: The osmolarity and viscosity of commonly used MR contrast agents

Trade name	*Osmolarity Osm/kg*	*Viscosity (cp)*
Gadodiamide	783	1.4
Gadopentetate dimeglumine	1960	2.9
Gadoteridol	630	1.3

and T2 increases. Signal will be decreased when hydrogen protons decrease, T1 increases or T2 decreases. CO_2, perfluorocarbons and deuterated water decrease protons as they possess no hydrogen nuclei. Paramagnetic materials like Gd, Fe and Mn decrease both T1 and T2 thereby altering the signal. Super paramagnetic particles reduceT2 thereby decreasing the signal. Diamagnetic substances have negative induced magnetization and are used in situations where they can displace or mix with normal tissue. Water, fat, perfluorocarbon and CO_2 are used as gastrointestinal contrast agents by the displacement of normal bowel contrast.

Contrast agents have been broadly classified as positive relaxation agents (T1 contrast agents) and negative relaxation agents (T2 contrast agents).

Positive Relaxation Agents

The contrast agent that affects T1 relaxation is referred as positive relaxation agent. These contrast agents reduce T1 relaxation times and shows increased signal intensity on T1 weighted images. The gadolinium chelates, namely paramagnetic agents, are examples of positive relaxation agents and have wide clinical application.

Negative Relaxation Agent

The contrast agent that affects T2 relaxation is referred to as negative relaxation agent. These contrast agents reduceT2 relaxation times resulting in decreased signal intensity on T2 weighted images. Examples of these contrast agents are ferromagnetic and supermagnetic metals. Gd chelates in high concentration can also be used as negative relaxation agents, provided fast imaging sequences are used. Perfusion imaging with high dose of contrast and associated EPI pulse technique reduces T2 with relative loss of signal.

Negative relaxation agents have a limited role in clinical practice.

Table: 9.2: Classification of contrast agents

Positive relaxation agents:

Parenteral (systemic):

- Gd-DTPA:Gadopentetatedimeglumine(magnevist)
- Gd-DTPA-BMA Gadodiamide(omniscan)
- Gd-HP-DO3A-Gadoteridol (prohance)
- Gd-BOPTA –Gadobenate dimeglumine

Gastrointestinal (oral):

- Gd-DTPA
- Ferric ammonium citrate(geritol)
- Vegetable oils, fats, etc.

Negative relaxation agents:

Parenteral (systemic):

- SPIO—Superparamagnetic iron oxide
- USPIO—Ultrasmall superparamagnetic iron oxide
- MION—Monocrystalline iron oxide

Gastrointestinal (oral):

- OMP—oral magnetic particles
- PFOB—Perfluoro octyl bromide

In post contrast images, the contrast enhancement is increased by various imaging parameters other than contrast media. Such parameters include magnetization transfer, fat suppression techniques, etc.

Magnetization Transfer (MT)

The application of magnetization transfer (MT) in spin echo imaging can improve the enhancement effect produced by a gadolinium chelate in the brain. MT pulses preferentially suppress the signal from background tissue, usually improving the conspicuity of gadolinium-enhanced regions. This can lead to improvement in the visualization of contrast enhancement at standard dose. Hence MT is advisable in all post contrast sequences in brain.

Fat Suppression

In areas of the body with abundant fat, T1 weighting with fat suppression (short T1 inversion recovery–STIR) provide improved depiction of contrast enhancement. Fat suppression is indicated in all fat rich areas like breast, retro-orbital and bone marrow, etc.

Perfusion Imaging

For perfusion imaging, the contrast medium is injected as a bolus using MRI compatible power injector. Images are acquired very rapidly during and immediately post injection. This helps to study the first pass of the contrast agent through the brain. In brain perfusion imaging studies T2 weighted scans are used. These scans provide the required high temporal resolution and are also quite sensitive to the vascular bed. On T2 weighted scans, the gadolinium chelates cause a reduction in signal intensity as opposed to the increase in signal intensity seen on T1 weighted scans. After acquisitions with the help of software relative cerebral blood volume (rCBV) and relative mean transit time (rMTT) of a given area is calculated. Perfusion imaging can detect brain ischemia far sooner than standard T2 weighted scans. It also detects the tissue at risk.

Administration of Contrast Agent

Administration of a gadolinium chelate can substantially improve lesion identification and characterization. After injection the MR contrast agent is distributed into the blood pool and extracellular fluid compartment of the body. In the brain lesion, enhancement occurs as a result of disruption of the blood brain barrier (BBB): MR contrast agents do not cross the normal blood brain barrier. The standard dose of gadolinium is 0.1 mmol/kg, which is equivalent to 0.2 ml/kg. The contrast is generally available in 10 or 20 ml vials. It is injected through the intravenous route and is rapidly excreted by glomerular filtration through the kidneys. Contrast agents have half-lives between 1 and 2 hours.

Adverse Reactions

There may be occasionally pain at the injection site. Nausea and vomiting are the two most common mild reactions encountered. Headache, paresthesia, dizziness, focal convulsions, skin reaction, flush are other adverse effects noted. There is no major change of incidence in various contrast agents regarding severe anaphylactoid reaction.

Patients with asthma, multiple allergies, or known drug sensitivity (including to iodinated contrast media) are at increased risk. The incidence of patients with adverse effects after IV injection of Gd-DTPA was found to be approximately 1 to 2%. In a post marketing survey of 5 million applications of Gd-DTPA, possible drug related death was reported in one patient. Gd contrast media are safe to be administered in children. During pregnancy use of contrast is not recommended as it crosses the placental barrier. Lactating mothers should stop breastfeeding their babies, as contrast is excreted in breast milk.

All emergency drugs should be made available while injecting contrast.

Hepatobiliary Agents

Gd-Benzyloxy propiomic tetraacetic acid (Gd-BOPTA) Multihance (Gadobenate dimeglumine) is used both in CNS and body. Multihance is excreted principally by the kidneys and to a small extent by the liver. The latter feature markedly improves the performance of this agent in the liver. Multihance binds to protein improving its relativity regardless of location in the body. Delayed scans are particularly useful for the detection of small liver metastases.

Feridex (fevumoxides, berlex laboratories) is a super paramagnetic iron oxide containing dextran, formulated for intravenous administration. This contrast agent is taken up by cells of the reticuloendothelial system (RES) and is sequestered by the RES, producing profound signal loss from normal background tissue. On T2 weighted images focal lesions like metastasis can be seen better. Its principal use is as a liver agent.

Tesla scan (Mn DPDP, Nycomed) agent was designed to be incorporated into hepatocytes. Post contrast moderate enhancement of normal liver parenchyma is seen improving lesion conspicuity.

Oral Contrast Agents

Complete bowel opacification is difficult and side effects are high due to the rapid transit of the agent through the bowel. The majority of the agents are eliminated rectally within the first few hours' administration and are not absorbed by the bowel. Either positive or negative relaxation agents can be used in bowel imaging. Positive contrast agents, increasing the signal intensity of the bowel are Gd-DTPA with a volume expander or ferric ammonium citrate (geritol). Examples of negative contrast agents, causing a reduction in signal intensity of the intestinal lumen, are small particles of iron oxide (SPIO-AMI-25) and ultrasmall particles of iron oxide (USPIO-AMI-227).

Magnetic resonance angiography can be performed with Gd contrast. After bolus injection of intravenous contrast a 10 to 20 fold reduction in blood T1 occurs during the first pass, producing a large signal between vessels and background tissue.

Tissue specific agents of MR contrast are yet to be standardized.

Conclusion

The gadolinium chelates play a major role as contrast agents in the evaluation of the patients by MRI. They improve sensitivity and specificity of the lesion detection.

Lesion delineation, assessment of lesion activity, and narrowing of differential diagnosis are improved with contrast study.

The MR contrast agents play an important role in routine practice. They are already stabilized in intracranial pathology and have improved the resolution in imaging of the vascular tree. Currently, new contrast agents are under development with the most promising being for liver imaging. Other contrast agents for bowel, lymph nodes and selective vascular imaging are yet to be standardized.

Ten

Recent Advances in Pulse Sequences

Magnetic resonance imaging (MRI) has created a new era in diagnosis and management of various diseases. Contrast in MRI is dependent on T1 relaxation, T2 relaxation and proton density. Depending on the predominant component, the image is called T1 weighted image, T2 weighted image or proton density (PD) image. The contrast is achieved by the basic pulse sequence namely, spin echo (SE), gradient recalled echo (GRE), and inversion recovery (IR). All the new pulse sequences have their origin in them.

The hydrogen protons present in the body act like tiny magnets. When the body is exposed to magnetic field the hydrogen protons align and precess. The precession frequency is proportional to the strength of the magnetic field. External energy in the form of Radiofrequency (RF) is applied to the precessing protons. There is disturbance in the magnetic equilibrium of the protons. Discontinuation of RF pulse causes the magnetic equilibrium of body to return to normal. While magnetic equilibrium is returning to normal it emits energy which is recorded as signal. It is the detected signal which forms the MR image.

Routine Sequences used in MRI

There are essentially three pulse sequences which are routinely used.

1. Spin echo (SE)
2. Inversion recovery (IR)
3. Gradient recalled echo (GRE) technique.

SPIN ECHO IMAGING

A spin echo sequence is the most commonly used technique in MRI.

A slice selection 90° RF pulse is applied in conjunction with a slice selection gradient. After a time of TE/2 a 180° slice selection gradient is applied. A phase encoding gradient is applied between the 90° and 180° pulses. The frequency encoding gradient is applied after the 180° pulse, during the time the signal is collected. The recorded signal is the echo (Fig. 10.1).

Repetition time (TR) is the time between successive excitation pulses for a given slice. Echo time (TE) is the time from the excitation pulse to the maximum echo.

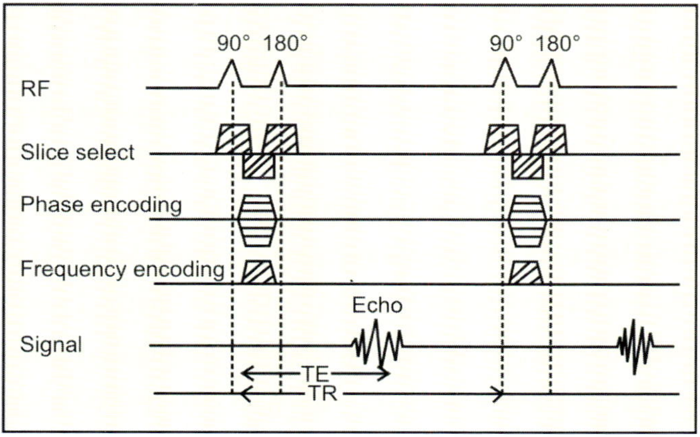

Fig. 10.1: Spin echo pulse sequence diagram

The contrast between white matter and edema is maximized in two distinct situations. A short repetition time (TR) and Echo time (TE) situation where white matter is brighter than edema and a long TR and TE situation where edema is brighter than white matter.

Gradients

The imaging plane or point is determined by applying magnetic field gradients. There are basically three types of gradient coils. One gradient is required in each of the x, y, and z direction. A gradient is simply a magnetic field that changes from point to point. Depending on their orientation axis they are called Gx, Gy, Gz, and used for slice select, frequency (read out), or phase encoding.

1. *Slice selection gradient*: It is turned on only during application of RF pulse. If we make the magnetic field change from point to point, then each position will have its own resonance frequency. We can make the magnetic field slightly weaker in strength at the feet and gradually increase in strength at the head. This effect is achieved by using slice selecting gradient coil. It helps to select the point of the slice.
2. *Phase encoding gradient*: The gradient is applied in one direction of the slice. Protons precess at slightly different speeds (according to the intensity of the gradient) and thus have different phase angles which make it possible to differentiate them. This operation is called phase encoding. Phase encoding gradient is usually applied between the 90° and the 180° RF pulses or between the 180° pulse and the echo. For every slice, each TR interval contains one phase encoding step. This

process completes one line in K-space corresponding to the selected gradient strength. This process is repeated to fill the entire K-space.

3. Frequency encoding gradient (read out gradient). This is applied perpendicular to the phase encoding. It gives rise to phase angle differences in each band of protons which previously had the same phase angle. The new phase angle provides spatial information. This operation is called frequency encoding. The frequency encoding gradient is applied during the time the echo is received, i.e. during read out. Each TR interval contains one read out per slice.

T1 and T2

T1 and T2 refer to physical properties of tissues after exposure to a series of pulses at predetermined time intervals. Different tissues have different T1 and T2 properties based on the response of their hydrogen nuclei to radiofrequency pulses imposed by the magnetic field. MRI exploits these different tissue properties by selecting equipment parameters (TE and TR) producing images based on either the T1 or T2 properties of the tissues. TE is the time interval between applying the pulse and receiving the signal. TR is interval between two radiofrequency pulses. TE and TR are both expressed in milliseconds (ms). A relatively low TE is about 20 ms, and high TE is above 100 ms. Low TR is about 50 ms and long TR is above 1500 ms T1 weighted images have a low TE and low TR (Fig. 10.2). Whereas both are high for T2 weighted images. Proton density images have a low TE and high TR (Fig. 10.3).

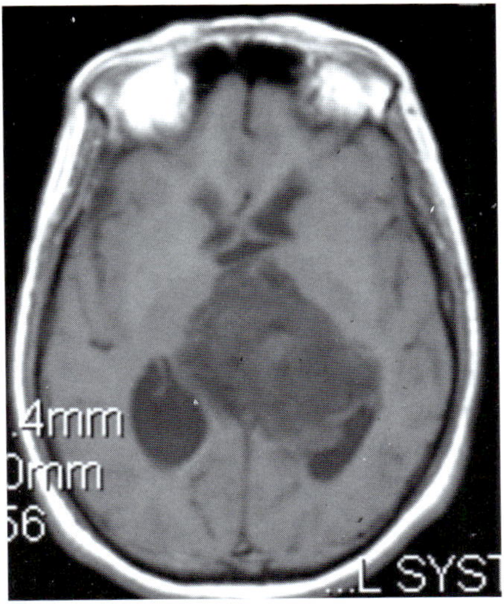

Fig. 10.2: Conventional spin echo T1 weighted image

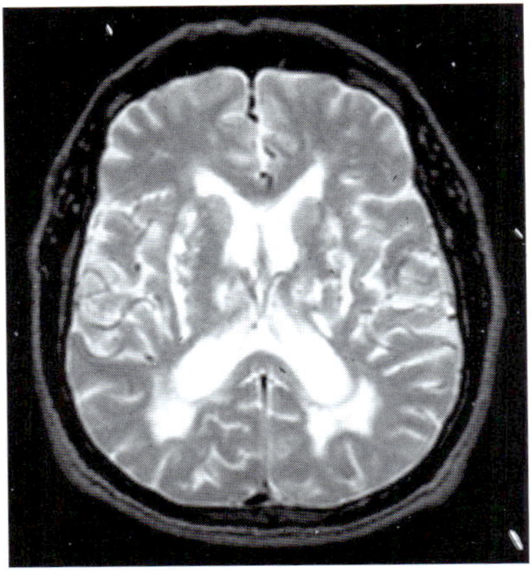

Fig. 10.3: Conventional spin echo T2 weighted image

CONTRAST

Contrast agent currently in use are paramagnetic substances. Molecules of paramagnetic contrast material create varying magnetic fields in tissues dependent on their vibration/tumbling velocities and concentration. These movements accelerate the relaxation process of the hydrogen nuclei in the tissues, shortening both T1 and T2. At certain tissue concentrations these substances produce a much shorter T1 effect and if image acquisition is T1 weighted certain tissues demonstrate contrast enhancement.

The most promising contrast material developed to date is Gd-DTPA (Gadolinium diethylenetriamine pentaacetic acid). It has a similar effect in MR as that of iodine in CT. However the action of gadolinium DTPA is to shorten T1 relaxation time and the area appears brighter on T1 weighted image (Fig. 10.4). In contrary the action of iodine in CT is to increase the density of area of the tissue and hence appears brighter.

INVERSION RECOVERY (IR)

The RF pulses are 180°–90°–180°. A slice selection 180° RF pulse is applied in conjunction with a slice selection

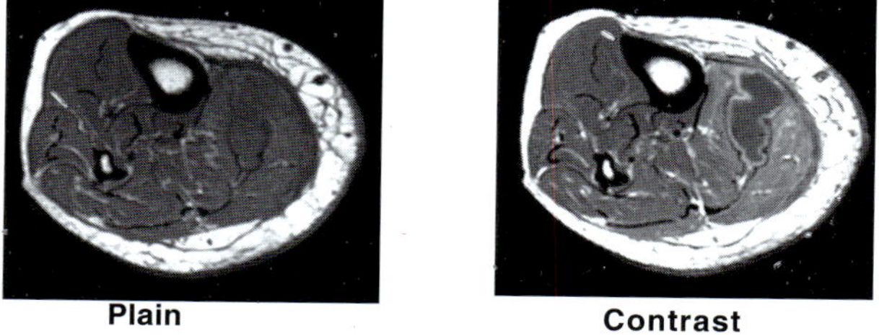

Fig. 10.4: Plain and contrast of calf showing enhancement of abscess

gradient. A period of time equal to inversion time (TI) elapses and a spin echo sequence is applied. The remainder of the sequence is equivalent to a spin echo sequence.

Inversion time (TI) is between the initial 180° pulse and 90° pulse. The inversion recovery sequence is generally used in a highly T1 dependent medium. Inversion recovery images are strongly T1 dependent providing excellent image contrast and anatomical details when the correct pulse parameters are used. Areas of short T1 appear bright (white) and areas of long T1 appear dark (black). Areas of low proton density such as cortical bone and air appear dark in IR sequence. Hence lesion adjacent to bone, e.g. Acoustic neuroma, chordoma, etc. cannot be easily distinguished (Fig. 10.5).

Short Inversion Time Inversion Recovery (STIR)

The T1 relaxation time of fat is 150 ms. By selection of inversion time (TI) equal to 150 ms, the fat in the images

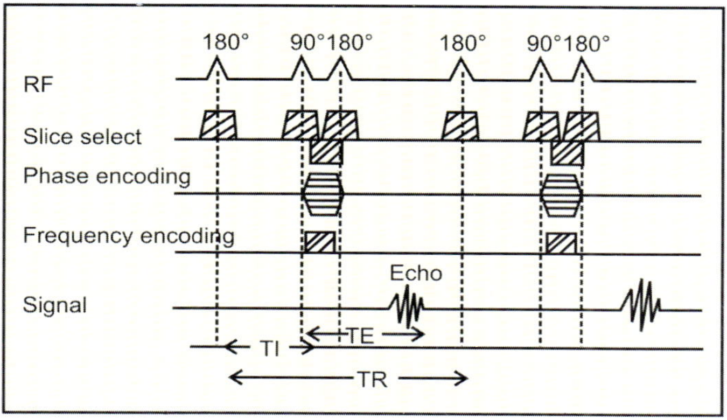

Fig. 10.5: Inversion recovery pulse sequence diagram

gets suppressed and it is termed as fat suppression images. This is useful technique in fatty tissues like retroorbital fat, musculoskeletal system and to differentiate between lipoma and subacute hematoma (methemoglobin stage) as both are hyperintense on T1 weighted images .Lipoma is a fatty lesion and is therefore suppressed on STIR sequences. The inversion time of 2000 ms suppresses CSF and it is known as FLAIR (Fluid attenuated inversion recovery).

FLAIR

Fluid attenuated inversion recovery (FLAIR) MR imaging techniques were first described by Hajnal et al.

In a IR sequence if the inversion time (TI) is increased to 1500 – 2000 msec the longitudinal magnetization of the brain is almost fully recovered. The signal from CSF can be nulled.

The FLAIR sequence has been used in the brain in cases of infarction and multiple sclerosis. The FLAIR sequence is used in heavily T2 weighted form in the brain where most lesions are highlighted . It also can be used to improve the accuracy of detecting T2 prolongation in the hippocampus in mesial temporal sclerosis. The CSF signal is decreased and this helps in detecting acute subarachnoid hemorrhage (Fig. 10.6).

One of the main disadvantages of FLAIR MR imaging was long acquisition times, however newer techniques combining FLAIR like sequences with fast spin echo techniques have greatly shortened acquisition times.

FLAIR technique is currently used in a variety of brain diseases including ischaemic stroke, demyelinating disorders, subarachnoid hemorrhage, meningitis, trauma (diffuse

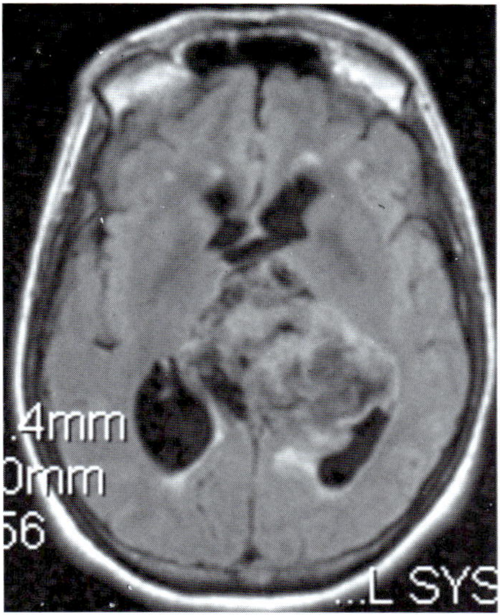

Fig. 10.6: FLAIR image

axonal injury), cystic lesions, tumors (pilocystic astrocytoma and glioblastoma multiforme) and vascular malformation.

Gradient Recalled Echo (GRE) Technique

Gradient echoes achieve their speed by using a low flip angle and gradient reversal resulting in a short TR. In GRE imaging sequence a slice selection RF pulse is applied to the imaged object. This RF pulse typically produces a rotation angle between 10 and 90 called flip angle. A refocusing gradient (read out direction) is employed that eliminates the original 180° pulse of SE and later recalls it at the echo time TE (hence the name gradient recalled echo or GRE (Fig. 10.7).

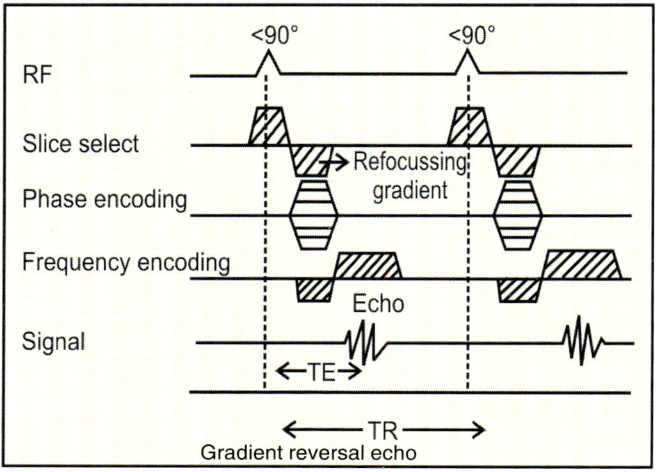

Fig. 10.7: Gradient reversal echo pulse diagram

Fast low angle shot (FLASH) and gradient recalled acquisition study state (GRASS) are examples of gradient echo technique. The shortening of TR values from seconds in conventional SE or IR sequences to tens of milliseconds in gradient echo sequences greatly reduces scan times.

The table below contains important acronyms used by major manufacturers.

Table 10.1: Important acronyms

GE	*SIEMENS*
GRASS	FISP
SPGR	FLASH
SSFP	PSIF
FSPGR	turbo-FLASH

GRASS	:	Gradient recalled acquisition in the steady state
SPGR	:	Spoiled GRASS
SSFP	:	Steady state free precession
FSPGR	:	Fast SPGR
FISP	:	Fast imaging with steady state precession
FLASH	:	Fast low angle shot
PSIF	:	Fast imaging with steady state precession (opposite of FISP)
Turbo-FLASH	:	(Turbo is used in place of Fast)

GRASS yields more T2* weighting images.

In SPGR, a long TR and a large a yield T1 weighting image. The disadvantages of SPGR include increased dephasing caused by inhomogeneity, increased magnetic susceptibility and chemical shift artifacts.

SSFP images yield heavily T2 (not T2*) weighted images with increased scan speed without the use of dedicated excitation and rephasing pulses. The advantages include decreased dephasing caused by inhomogeneity, decreased magnetic susceptibility and chemical shift artifacts. The disadvantages are decreased SNR and increased sensitivity to nonstationary tissue.

Multiplanar Techniques: The GRASS and SPGR sequences can be performed using a multiplanar technique by selecting a long TR. These are called MPGR (multiplanar gradient recalled, MPSPGR. A small α yields PD weighted while a large α yields T1 weighting. Advantages of multiplanar technique include increased SNR, mutiplanar scanning, multiecho imaging and reduces saturation effects.

Fast Gradient Echo Technique: The GRE techniques are generally faster than SE techniques. There are additional methods to increase the speed of scanning. These methods are called Fast GRASS, Fast SPGR Fast multiplanar GRASS, Fast multiplanar spoiled GRASS, etc. Ultrafast TRs and TEs are employed to reduce the sequence time. This is achieved by fractional echo, fractional RF, fractional NEX, and reduction in the sampling time (increasing the band width).

Advantages of Fast GRE Techniques

1. Single breath hold techniques in the abdomen.
2. Imaging a joint in motion.
3. Cine imaging of the heart.
4. Temporal scanning of the same slices after contrast administration.
5. Perfusion imaging.

Disadvantages of Fast GRE

1. Decreased SNR
2. Increased chemical shift artifacts.

FLOW IMAGING

GRE scanning performs one slice at a time except in multiplanar imaging. Each slice is an entry slice. Consequently, flow related enhancement (FRE) applies to every single slice, and vessels appear bright on GRE images. No saturated flowing protons enter the slice, so that flipping these protons yields maximum signal. This is the basic concept behind 2D or 3D Time of Flight (TOF) MR angiography.

RAPID SCAN TECHNIQUES

As a result of ongoing technical developments rapid scan techniques have established themselves as indispensable for state of the art clinical magnetic resonance imaging. A ten minute scan protocol is becoming popular for most of the routine imaging. Rapid MR techniques are based on either gradient recalled or RF refocusing.

Radiofrequency Refocussed Technique

This achieves speed by sampling multiple lines of K space per TR. Fast spin echo (FSE), Turbo spin echo (TSE) and Half Fourier Single Shot Turbo Spin Echo (HASTE) are the examples of this technique.

FAST SPIN ECHO

In fast spin echo (FSE) long train of RF focusing pulses can be applied to create multiple SE's after an initial RF excitation pulse, then the individual echoes may be differently phase encoded to produce a data set for image reconstruction. This principle underlines the RARE (rapid acquisition with relaxation enhancement) imaging technique.

Fast spin echo (FSE) is one of the most important recent advances in MRI. It was originally called RARE. The primary advantages of FSE is speed without the usual concomitant loss of signal to noise ratio (Fig. 10.8).

The essential difference between convential spin echo (CSE) and FSE is that in CSE all echoes in a train are preceded by a single value of phase encoding gradient whereas in FSE each echo in a train is preceded by different value of the phase encoding gradient (Fig. 10.9).

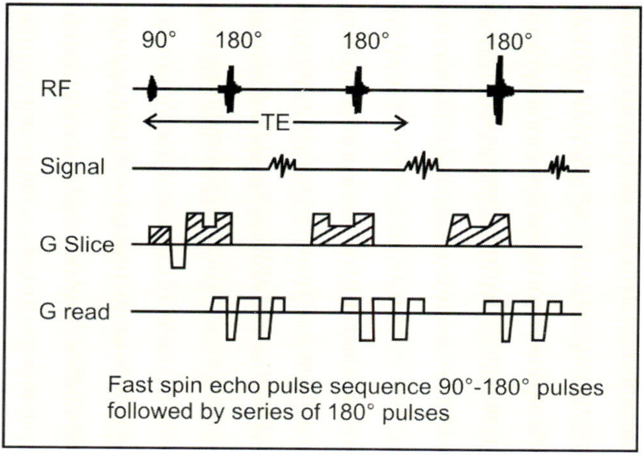

Fig. 10.8: Fast spin echo pulse sequence diagram

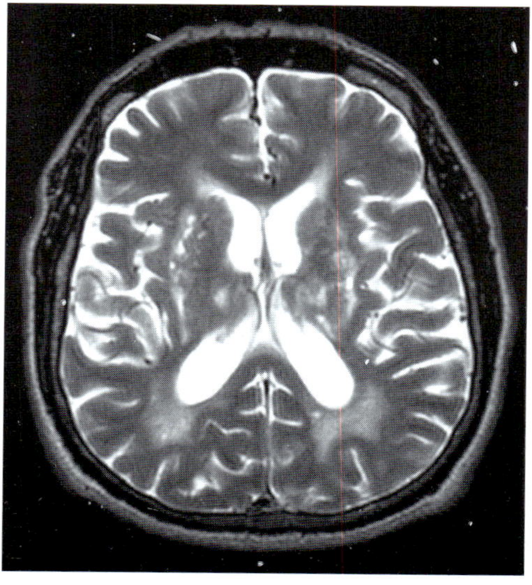

Fig. 10.9: Fast spin echo T2 weighted image

For an eight echo train length the scan time is reduced by a factor of 8. FSE can use a higher TR, larger matrix and is more advantageous than CSE and still do it in much reduced times (Fig. 10.10).

Fast spin echo advantages include acquisition of true T2 weighted images and the possibility of thin section T2 weighted three-dimensional imaging. FSE is relatively insensitive to magnetic susceptibility effects hence artifacts produced by metallic objects are reduced. However, small hemorrhagic or calcified lesions may be missed. Fat is bright on proton density and T2 weighted images on FSE compared to CSE.

Subtle differences between FSE and CSE imaging include failure to detect small objects with T2 values close to background, minor changes in the size of small objects, and decreased signal in some stationary tissues related to increased magnetization tranfer and saturation effects in fast SE images. The protein bound water is relatively suppressed on FSE images compared with CSE images.

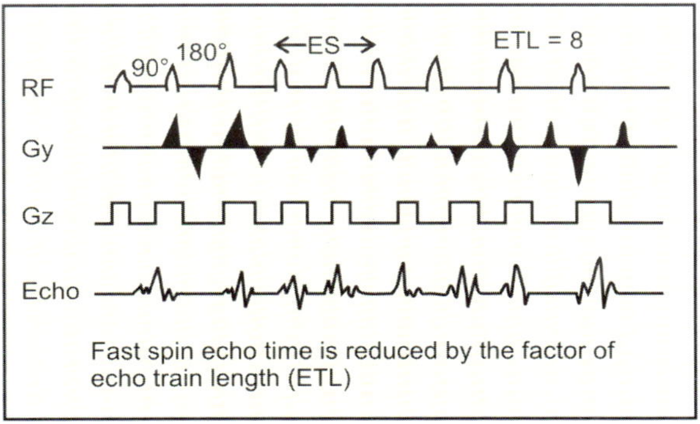

Fig. 10.10: Fast spin echo T2 weighted image

This effect is most noticeable in the spine where normally hydrated disks are bright on T2 weighted CSE images but some what darker on FSE images.

In general FSE sequences have replaced CSE sequences for many clinical applications because they provide a comparable signal to noise ratio (SNR) and image contrast at significantly shorter scan times.

Half Fourier imaging uses only about half the number of phase encoding steps of conventional image matrix. For example, a K-space consists of 256 horizontal lines with 256 data samples with a spatial resolution of 256 * 256 pixels. Imaging times may be cut by a factor of 2 if only half of the data in K-space is acquired saving 50 percent in imaging time.

ECHOPLANAR IMAGING

Echoplanar imaging fills K-space after a single RF pulse in a single measurement or shot.

A magnetic resonance image is referred to as image space. Its Fourier transform is referred to as K-space. In magnetic resonance imaging K-space is equivalent to the space defined by the frequency and phase encoding directions. Conventional imaging sequences record one line of K-space in each encoding step. Since one phase encoding step occurs with each TR time, the time required to produce an image is determined by the product of TR and the number of phase encoding steps. Echoplanar imaging measures all lines of K-space in a single TR period.

There is a 90° slice selection RF pulse which is applied in conjunction with a slice selection gradient. There is an initial phase encoding gradient pulse. Next there is 180°

pulse. There are 128 or 256 phase and frequency encoding gradients when the echo is recorded. The rate at which K-space is reversed is rapid (Fig. 10.11).

The greatest application of echoplanar imaging appears to be in the area of functional MRI of the brain. During brain activity there is a rapid momentary increase in the blood flow to the specific thought center in the brain. Similarly, movement of index finger causes rapid momentary increase in the circulation of the specific part of the brain controlling the movement of the finger. The increase in oxygen (which is paramagnetic) affects the T1 and T2 of the local brain tissues. The difference in T1 and T2 relative to surrounding tissue causes a contrast between the tissues. This is known as BOLD (blood oxygen level detection) technique (Fig. 10.12).

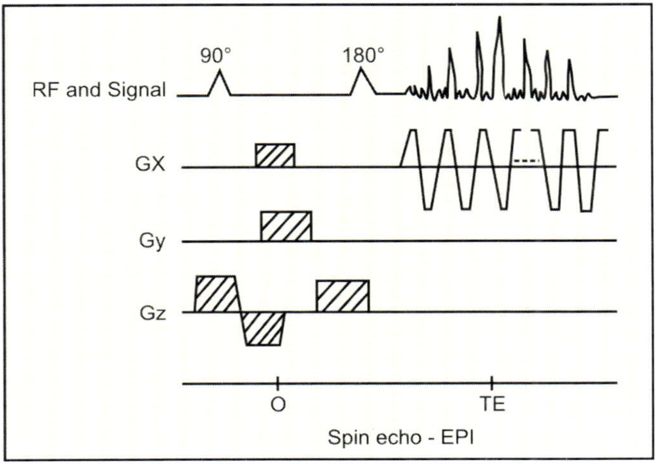

Fig. 10.11: Spin echo- EPI pulse sequence diagram

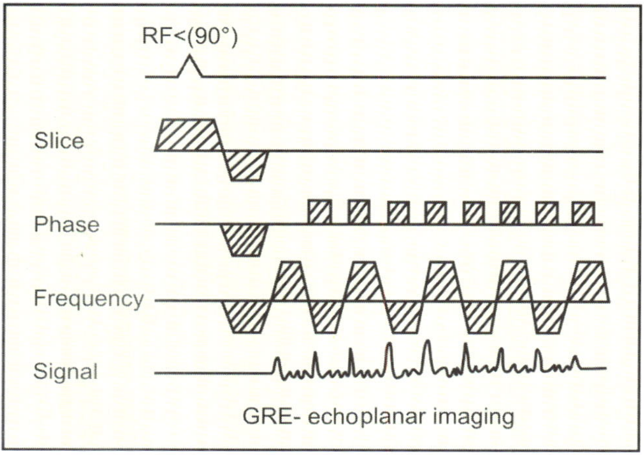

Fig. 10.12: GRE-EPI pulse sequence diagram

ECHOPLANAR DIFFUSION IMAGING

Diffusion imaging is accomplished by adding diffusion sensitizing gradient pulses on either side of the 180° of a SE sequence either CSE or SE-EPI.

Diffusion is the process of random thermal motion of molecules (Brownian motion). These motions occur at microscopic scale (i.e. on the order of tenths or hundredths of millimeter per second). To enable MR acquisition to detect these small motions, gradients applied across the imaging field gradients, experience a phase change. These phase changes either combine to retain signal, or combine to reduce signal. Signal loss is related to the product of the apparent diffusion coefficient of the tissue and b value of the sequence, which is determined by the amplitude, duration and spacing of the additional gradient pulses (Fig. 10.13).

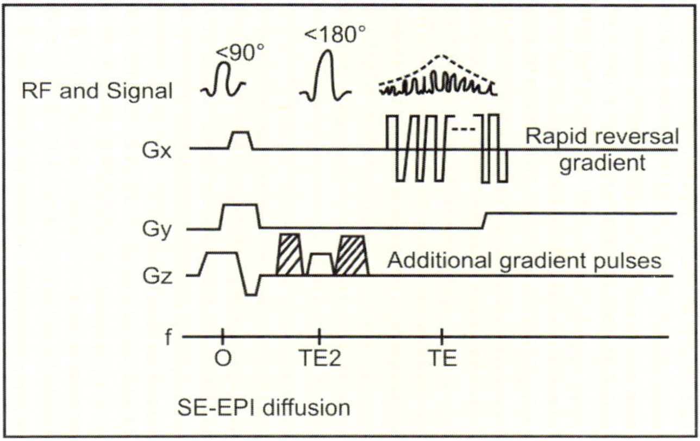

Fig. 10.13: Spin echo EPI diffusion

In echoplanar diffusion imaging of the brain two or more acquisitions must be made. First a base line SE-EPI image is made with the diffusion sensitizing gradient off (b=0) establishing a reference image. Next a diffusion sensitized image is taken using a b value in the range of 1000 sec/ mm^2. Typically the following four sequences are required: b=0 baseline image and then b=1000 images sensitizing along each of the three (x, y and z) axes. In each diffusion image white matter tracts running parallel to the gradients appear dark and white matter tracts running perpendicular to the gradients appear bright reflecting the preferred diffusion direction of water along the axons (Fig. 10.14).

Because this bright signal can potentially simulate pathology (i.e. ischemic lesion), lesions must be assessed in all three diffusion images to accurately diagnose pathology. Alternatively a trace image can be acquired showing the average diffusion changes along the three axes.

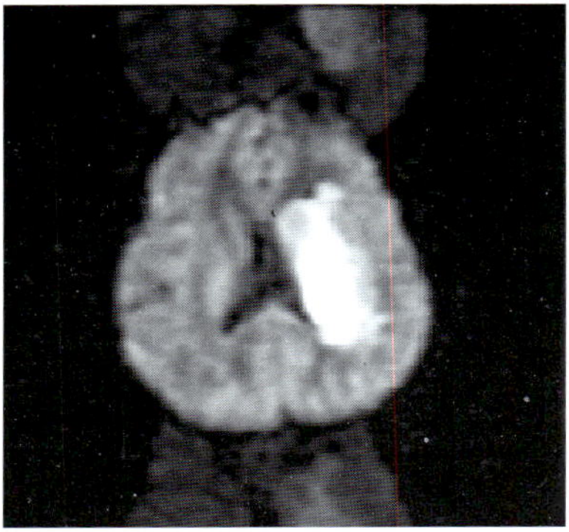

Fig. 10.14: Diffusion image

ECHOPLANAR PERFUSION IMAGING

Perfusion or blood flow of the brain can be assessed with EPI by monitoring the first pass effect of gadolinium contrast. T2 weighted EPI sequences can be used to measure susceptibility changes caused by the passage of the paramagnetic contrast agent. Large macromolecules of gadolinium do not cross the blood brain barrier. As this bolus traverses vascular bed it changes the intravascular signal and dephases spins outside the lumen in the nearby tissues. This long range intravascular phenomenon has the beneficial effect of increasing the potential volume of tissue signal changes.

The transient drop in the signal intensity caused by the passage of the gadolinium bolus provides indirect evidence of the state of perfusion of the tissue. From these data, relative cerebral blood volume (rCBV) and mean transit time (MTT) maps can be generated. The sensitivity to perfusion in vessels of a particular site depends on the specific EPI sequence used. Performing echoplanar perfusion imaging with a spin echo (SE-EPI) provides sensitivity to the microcirculation alone and a GRE-EPI sequence provides sensitivity to both the microcirculation and the capillary circulation (Fig. 10.15).

MAGNETIZATION TRANSFER CONTRAST (MTC)

The main use of MTC is to extract more information from relaxation of biological tissues. In most biological tissue, there is cross relaxation between the free proton pool in protons in moving water (Hf) and the restricted proton pool in protons in stationary water or tissues such as macromolecues (Hr).

Only protons that have a sufficiently long T2 time (Hf) can be imaged. Typically, these protons are found in moving water. Other protons (Hr) lose their transverse magnetization decay before their signal is collected.

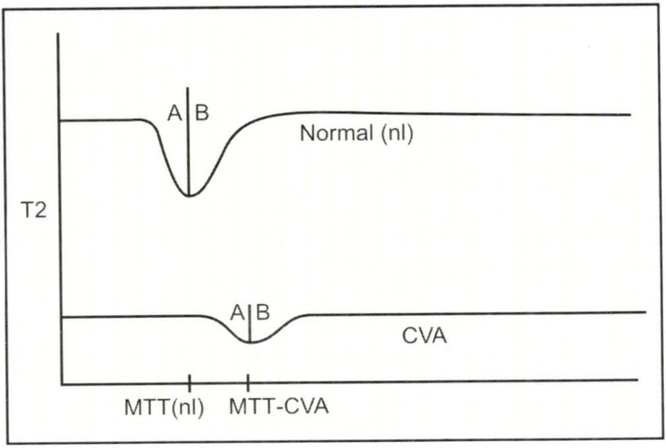

Fig. 10.15: Echoplanar perfusion graph

Magnetization is constantly being transferred between Hf and Hr and this will result in a change to the T1 values of Hf. If the Hr pool is saturated by off resonance irradiation, this will reduce its magnetization to zero. This causes loss of signal intensity from the Hf pool at the interface between the two pools. Due to the very short T2 value of the Hr pool, the behavior of the magnetization during the RF pulse is dominated by relaxation. Hr makes up only around 10 percent of the total proton pool in muscle tissue and therefore continuous or repeated saturation is needed to create sufficient MTC in the Hf pool. MTC is particularly good at increasing the T1 contrast between normal and diseased tissue and is noted as being particularly useful in MR angiography.

MTC is proposed by most MRI manufacturers as a standard push button technique. It has been widely applied in clinical routines. Main applications are the suppression of background tissue in MR angiography, and synergetic enhancement of contrast in the T2 weighted or contrast agent enhanced scans.

However, only recently has the value of MTC for assessing tissue diseases by quantitative indexes started to emerge.

MAGNETIC RESONANCE OF ANGIOGRAPHY (MRA)

Magnetic resonance angiography is a noninvasive method of study of blood vessels. Fast imaging techniques like gradient echo are used for MRA. There are two major ways of performing MRA (i) Time of Flight (TOF), (ii) Phase Contrast (PC).

TIME OF FLIGHT

In TOF angiography low flip angle is used and 180° pulse is eliminated. Stationary tissue is exposed to multiple RF pulses and is fully saturated. Unsaturated blood entering this slice gives high signal. Obviously, maximum enhancement will be obtained when the imaging plane is at right angles to the direction of blood flow (Figs 10.16 and 10.17).

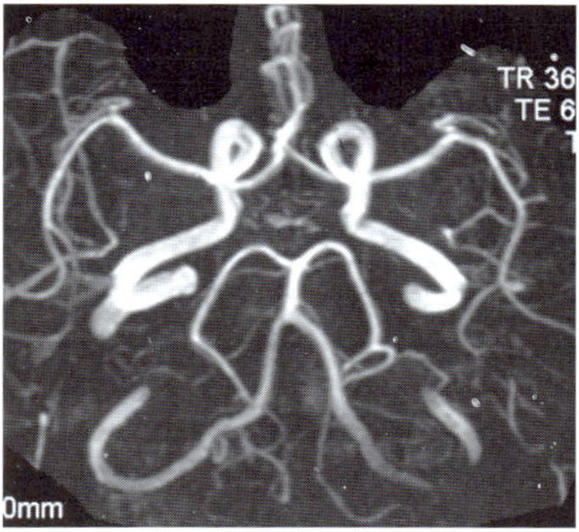

Fig. 10.16: MR angiography TOF technique. Circle of Willis

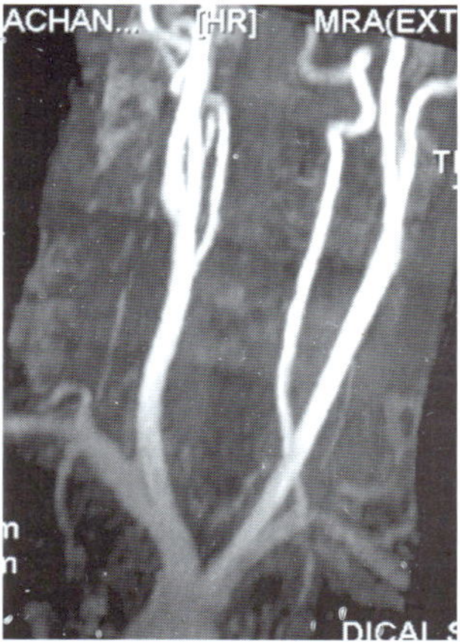

Fig. 10.17: MR angiography TOF technique extracranial vessels

PHASE CONTRAST

PC MRA is based on the principle that flow of blood along a magnetic field gradient causes a phase shift in the MR signal. Pairs of images are obtained using different gradient polarities. One image of a pair will be obtained with a gradient of positive polarity to induce positive flow related phase shift, whilst for the other image a gradient of negative polarity is used to induce a negative flow related phase shift. These images are subtracted to delete stationary tissue so that only blood vessels are seen. Phase contrast sequences have to be encoded for specific peak velocities. Unlike multiple projection images on TOF MRA, in PC MRA a single collapsed image available from the subtracted phase,forms the source image (Fig. 10.18).

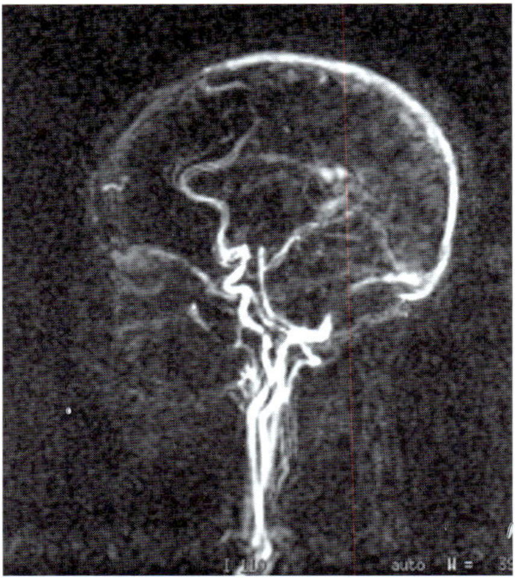

Fig. 10.18: MR venography PC technique dural sinuses

Table 10.2: TOF versus phase contrast

	TOF	*PC*
Images	Multiple projection	Usually single collapsed
Bright Met Hb	Simulates flow	Image subtracted
Slice thickness	1-2 mm	3-5 mm
Resolution	Good	Fair
Flow sensitivity	Fair	Good
Time	3-4 min	7-8 min

Table 10.3: MR angiography clinical application

Method	***Anatomy***
1. 2 D TOF	(Conventional carotid artery overview, venous flow gradient echo)
2. 3 D TOF with MOTSA	Carotid artery overview with optimal visualization of stenosis. Combined with contrast for intracranial aneurysm
3. 3 D TOF with MOTSA and MTC	Cerebral arteries dural sinus (< 20 cm/s)
4. 2 D PCA	Vertebral basilar system (30 cm/s)
5. 3 D PCA	Carotid arteries (30-60 cm/s)

MR SPECTROSCOPY

MR Spectroscopy (MRS) relies on information provided by chemical shifts. The magnetic field around nuclei in a chemically complex environment is altered due to shielding currents that are associated with the electron distribution around adjacent atoms. These alterations in the magnetic field cause small changes in the resonance frequency which are known as chemical shifts and these allow a distinction to be made between the small nuclei in different chemical environment.

MR spectroscopy may be obtained with many clinical 1.5 T MR units. Adequate MR spectra may be obtained in periods of time as short as 10 to 15 minutes. Therefore, they may be added to routine MR imaging studies. MR spectroscopy provides greater information concerning tissue characterization than what is possible with MR imaging studies alone.

31P MR spectroscopy can be utilized to measure the concentration of ATP, phosphocreatine and inorganic phosphate as well as the intracellular pH in muscle. The metabolites of interest in brain include N-acetyle aspartate (NAA), choline containing compounds (Cho) as well as creatine and phosphocreatine (Cr). The NAA serves as a marker of neurons. In a variety of disorders it may be decreased where there is little or no change on the MR image (Fig. 10.19).

Proton spectroscopy appears complementary to MR imaging which generally of value in acute and subacute disease. Proton MR spectroscopy readily distinguishes normal brain from tissues from astrocytoma. However,

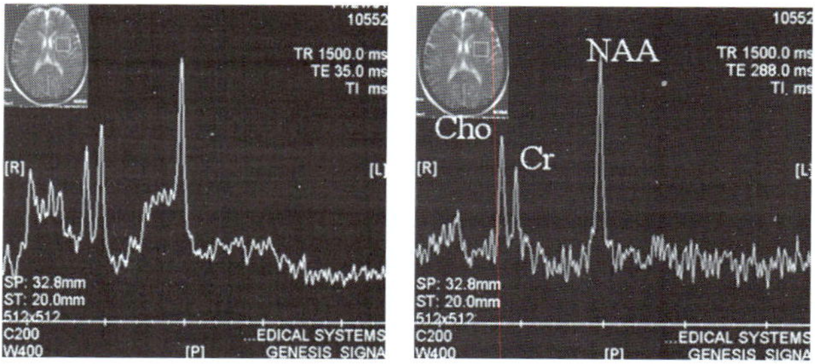

TE 35 TE 288

Fig. 10.19: MR spectroscopy

proton MR spectroscopy may not be able to distinguish between different histologic grades of malignancy in astrocytoma. MR spectroscopy may be useful in difficult cases to differentiate tumors. Proton MR spectroscopy shows elevation of lactate in patients who have received 40 Gy or more to the brain. It also demonstrates marked metabolic alterations in patients with mild AIDS related dementia. Spectroscopy is also helpful in degenerative disorders like Alzheimer and Parkinson disease, hepatic encephalopathy, cerebral ischaemia, etc. some innovative applications include measurment of psychoactive drugs, neurofibromatosis type 1, cerebral heterotopias, multiple sclerosis, etc.

CONCLUSIONS

Rapid scanning techniques have established themselves as indispensable for state-of art clinical magnetic resonance imaging. A major breakthrough came with introduction of low flip angle gradient echo imaging which is the basis for most recent advances. Now we have magnets with high field strengths (1.5T – 3T) high gradient strength 25-40 mt/m which enables far better contrast functional imaging. MR spectroscopy is a new development and its application in metabolic and functional imaging is rapidly evolving. Recent advances in MRI include new pulse sequences, rapid scanning, functional imaging, angiography and spectroscopy.

Eleven

Practical Imaging

IMAGE PRESENTATION

Each displayed image will have two orientation labels, one at the top, and the other at the left of the image. Images from the three standard orthogonal planes are displayed in the following manner in the absence of a scout:

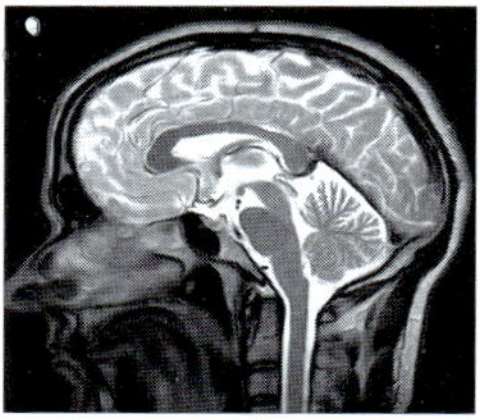

Fig. 11.1

Sagittal Images: These are displayed with the patient's anterior to the left (marked A), and the superior portion of the image (marked S) at the top of the screen. Slices are numbered and displayed sequentially, beginning on the patient's right and proceeding leftward.

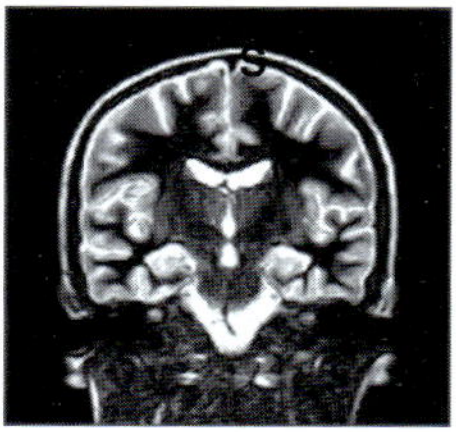

Fig. 11.2

Coronal Images: These are displayed with the patient's right side (marked R) on the left side of the screen. The superior portion of the image is at the top of the screen (marked S). The slices are numbered and displayed sequentially from posterior to anterior.

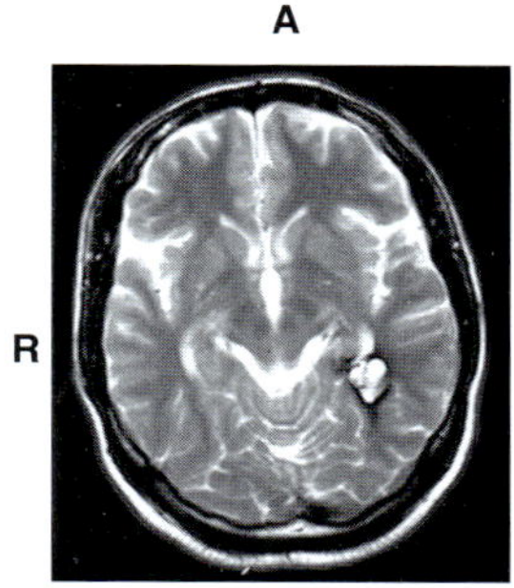

Fig. 11.3

Axial Images: These are displayed with the patient's right side (marked R) on the left side of the screen and the anterior portion of the image at the top of the screen (marked A). Slices are numbered and displayed from inferior to superior.

SCOUT SLICE PLACEMENT AND ANGLES

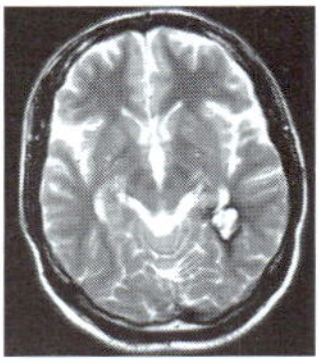

Using an axial scout

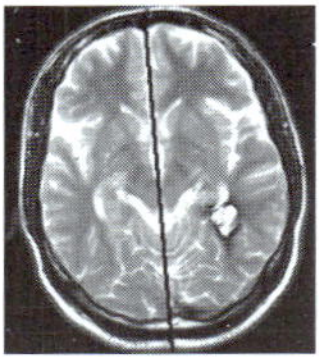

Allows only a sagittal image

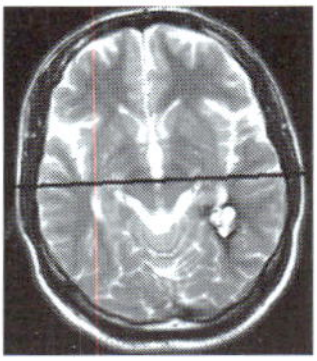

Allows only a coronal image

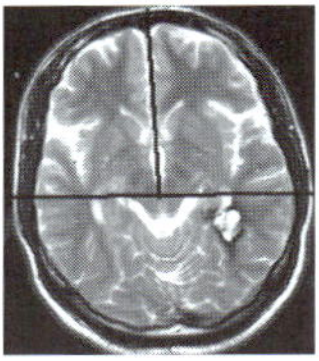

Allows obliquing for rotation

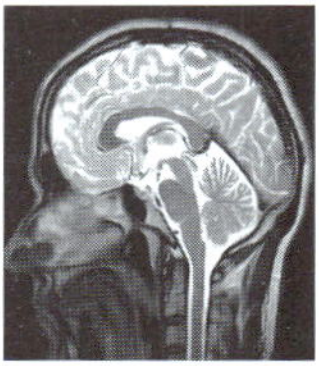

Using an sagittal scout

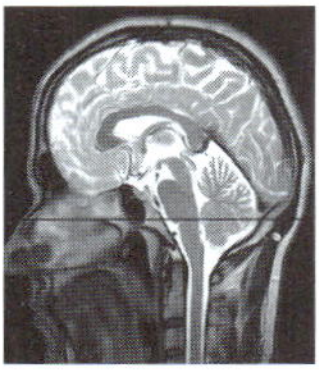

Allows only an axial image

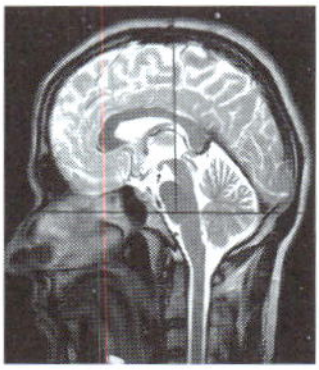

Allows obliquing for rotation

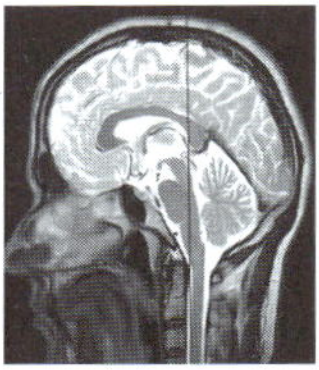

Allows only coronal image

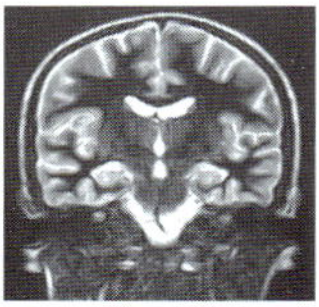

Using a coronal scout

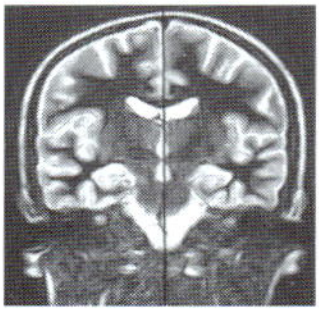

Allows only a sagittal image

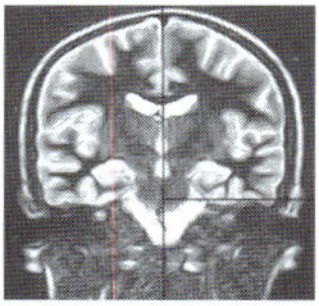

Allows obliquing for rotation

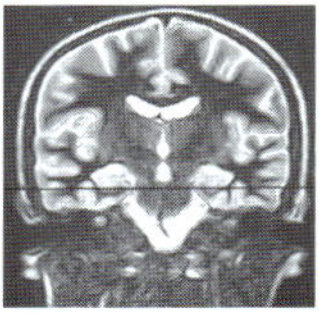

Allows only an axial image

IMAGE REVIEW

Identifying Image Labels

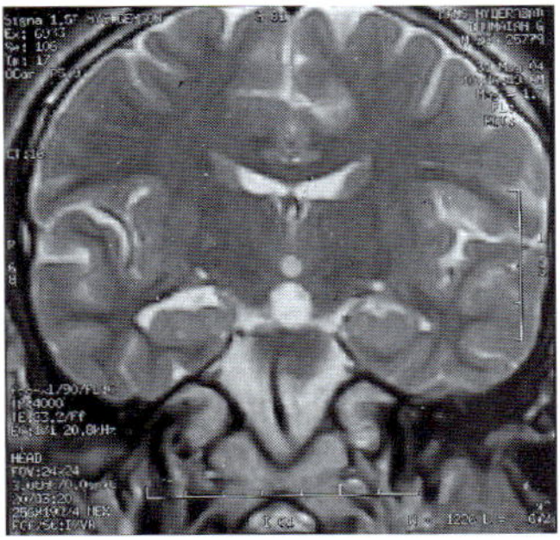

Fig. 11.16

Right

Signa 1.5 T	: Equipment name
Se	: Series number
Im	: Image Nnmber
OAX	: Plane sequence
ET	: Echo train length
R/L	: Side orientation marks
S/I	: Top orientation marks
TR	: Repetition time
TE	: Echo time
31.2	: Band width
Head	: Coil name
FOV	: Field of view
	: Thickness and spacing
	: No. of slice and acquisition time
	: Frequency and phase encoding matrix
N ex	: Number of excitations
F Cf	: Flow compensation
NP	: No phase wrap
VB	: Variable bandwidth

Left

NIMS Hyderabad	: Institution name and place
	: Patient name
	: Gender, age and IP number
	: Date
	: Time
Mag	: Magnification
FL	: Filter
ROT	: Rotation
W	: Window width
L	: Window level
ν	: Frequency encoding
	: Measurement scale in mm

ANATOMICAL REFERENCE POINTS

The following anatomical reference points are provided as a general guideline for patient positioning. Internal structures of the body may be located at different positions depending on patient size. When you are not sure of the exact location of the area of interest, use the standard protocols provided at your site, and perform a scout scan.

Head protocol—align red cross with orbital/meatal line

Breast protocol—align red cross with nipple line

Chest protocol—align red cross with mid-sternum

Abdomen protocol—align red cross with twelfth rib

Pelvic scan—align red cross with anterior superior iliac spine (ASIS)

The chart below provides reference points for common anatomical structures.

Anatomical level	Reference points
C-1	Mastoid Tip (most inferior level of skull). Coincides with foramen magnum
C-3	Hyoid Bone
C-5, C-6	Thyroid Cartilage
C-7	Level of Shoulder, Vertebral Prominence
T-1	1.5 Inches(3.8 cm) superior to suprasternal notch
T-2, T-3	Suprasternal Notch
T-4, T-5	Sternal Angle, Second Costal Cartilage
T-7	3 inches (7.6 cm) inferior to Sternal Angle
T-9, T-10	Xiphoid Tip
L-3	Bottom of Ribs
L-3, L-4	Iliac Crest, Umbilicus

L-5, S-1	Midway between iliac crest and Anterior Superior Iliac Supine
S-2	Anterior Superior Iliac Supine
Skull Base	Mastoid Tip
Pituitary(Sella Turcica)	1.5 inches (3.8 cm) Anterior and Superior to External Auditory Meatus
Orbits	Orbital-Meatal (OM) Line
Heart(Superior Border)	T-4, T-5, Sternal Angle
Heart [Inferior (Apex)]	Fifth or Sixth Rib
Kidneys	T-12 through L-3 (Right Kidney is higher.)
Gallbladder	T-9-Xiphoid Tip
Pancreas	Xiphoid Tip
Bladder	Symphysis Pubis

MRI EXAMINATIONS BY ANATOMICAL REGION

HEAD AND NECK

1. Brain
2. Temporal Lobes
3. Posterior Fossa and IAM
4. Pituitary
5. Orbits
6. T-M Joint
7. Diffusion
8. Perfusion
9. Spectroscopy
10. Functional
11. MRA-Head
12. MRV
13. MRI in Steriotaxy
14. D.B.S
15. CSF-Flow
16. CSF-Rhinorrhea
17. MRA Neck

SPINE

18. C-Spine
19. D-Spine
20. L-Spine
21. Whole Spine

CHEST AND ABDOMEN

22. Chest

23. Heart and great vessels
24. Breast
25. Brachial Plexus
26. Abdominal Angio
27. MRCP
28. MRU
29. Pelvis
30. Endorectal

UPPER EXTREMITY

31. Shoulder
32. Humerus
33. Elbow
34. Forearm
35. Wrist and Hand

LOWER EXTREMITY

36. Hips
37. Thigh
38. Knee Joint
39. Tibia and Fibula
40. Ankle
41. Vascular Imaging

HEAD AND NECK

BRAIN

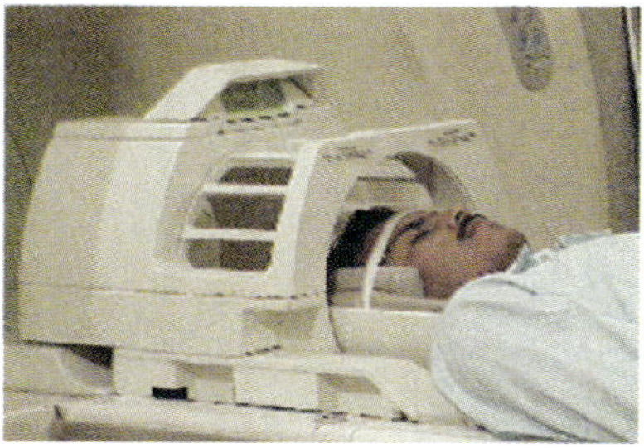

Patient Position-Head coil

Patient Position-Head coil:
- Set-up the head coil
- Place the patient in the head coil
- Immobilize the patient using sponges and straps

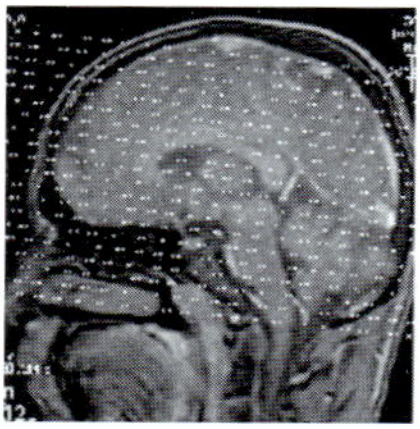

Sagittal localizer to obtain axial slices

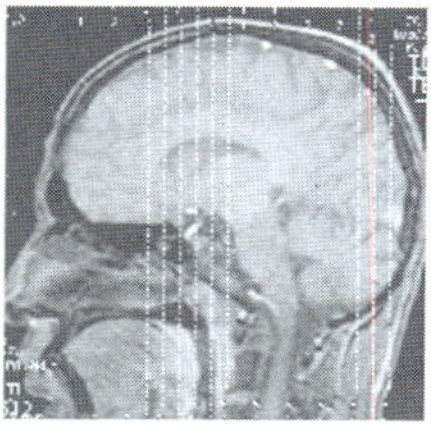

Sagittal localizer to obtain coronal slices

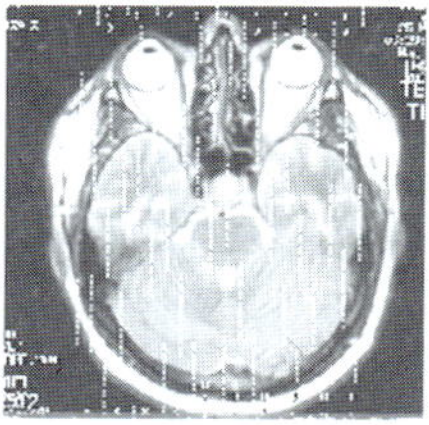

Axial localizer to obtain sagittal slices

BRAIN

Indication

- Evaluation of infarction , AIDS
- Multiple sclerosis(MS), Primary tumor assessment and metastatic disease
- Unexplained neurological symptoms or deficit

Sequences

Pulse Sequence	Axial T2 FSE	Axial T1 FSE	Axial T1 SE	Sag T2 FSE	Cor T2 FSE	Axial Flair
TR	4900	525	600	3650	4000	9000
TE/IR	85	Min.	Min.	85	85	120/2000
ETL	16	2	—	15	15	—
Bandwidth	20.83	20.83	20.83	20.83	20.83	15.63
Nex	2	1	2	2	2	1
Slice	5	5	5	5	5	5
Gap	1.5	1.5	1.5	1	1.5	1.5
No. of Slices	20	20	20	20	20	20
Matrix Freq/Phase	256 / 256	256 / 256	512/256	256 / 256	256 / 256	256/192
FOV	24	24	24	24	24	24
SNR	100	100	100	100	100	100
Scan Time	2.02	1.44	3.54	2.18	2.00	4.12
Frequency Direction	A/P	A/P	A/P	S/I	S/I	A/P
Auto Center Frequency	Water	Water	Water	Water	Water	Water
Flow Compensation Direction	Slice	—	—	Freq	Freq	Slice
Saturation	I	I	I	I	I	I

Contrast Usage: Inject Gadolinium (10 ml), if pathological conditions seen. Acquire post-contrast T1W Images in all 3 planes

TEMPORAL LOBES

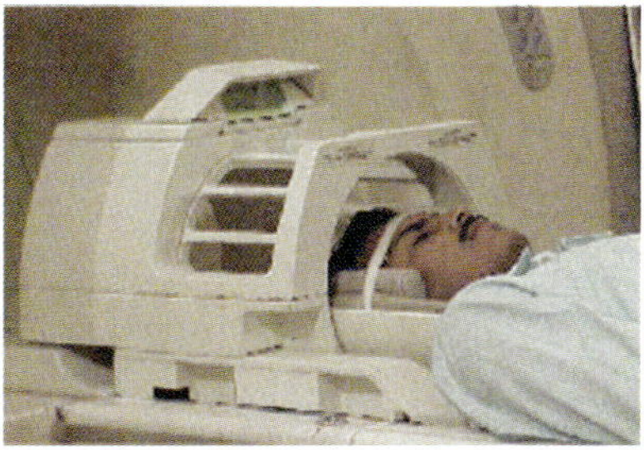

Patient Position-Head coil

- Set-up the head coil
- Place the patient in the head coil
- Immobilize the patient using sponges and straps

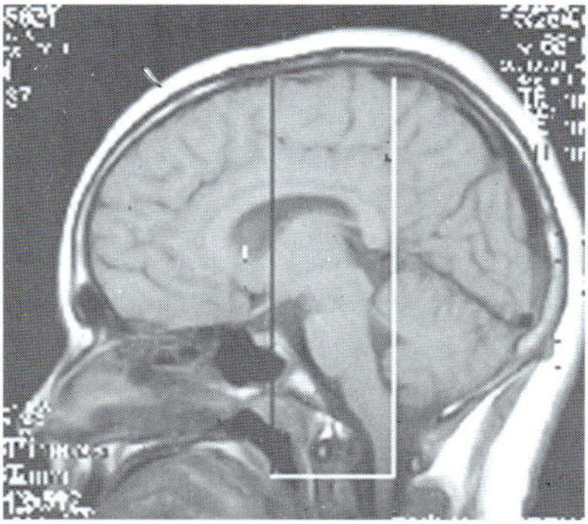

Sagittal localizer to obtain coronal slices of the hippocampus

PROTOCOL: TEMPORAL LOBES

Indication

- Diagnosis and evaluation of a lesion specifically in the temporal lobes (tumours, vascular malformation, leukodystrophies and atrophic processes).
- Evaluation of signal change in the hippocampus and the temporal lobe.
- Measurements of the hippocampal volume (hippocampal atrophy is presently considered the most sensitive indicator of hippocampal disease).

Sequences

Pulse Sequence	Axial T2	Oblique Cor T1	Oblique Cor T2	Oblique Cor-FLAIR	Cor 3DSPGR
TR	4900	400	4000	4200	30
TE/IR	85	Min	85	50/350	Min
ETL	16	2	16	12	FA-45 Deg.
Bandwidth	20.83	20.83	15.63	20.83	15.63
Nex	2	4	4	2	2
Slice	5	4	4	4	1.5
Gap	1.5	1	1	1	No. of scan locs: 28
No. of Slices	20	16	16	16	Slab 1
Matrix Freq/Phase	256/256	256/192	320/256	320/192	256/192
FOV	24	16	16	16	20
SNR	100	65	100	94	100
Scan Time	2.02	5.12	4.24	4.37	6.12
Frequency Direction	A/P	S/I	S/I	S/I	S/I
Auto Center Frequency	Water	Water	Water	Water	Water
Flow Compensation Direction	Slice	——	Freq	Freq	——
Saturation	I	I	I	I	I

INTERNAL AUDITORY MEATUS

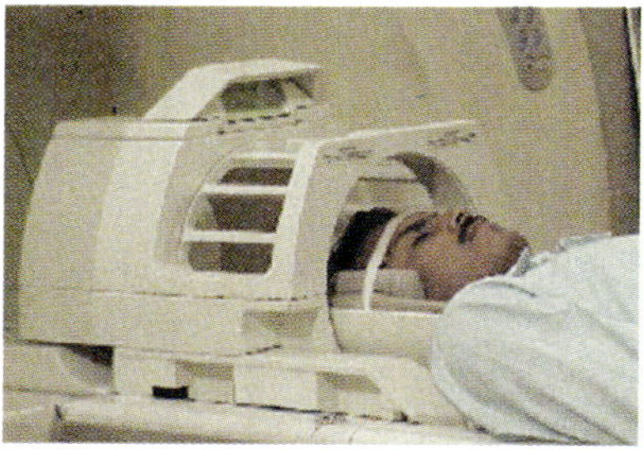

Patient Position-Head Coil

Patient Position-Head coil:
- Set-up the head coil
- Place the patient in the head coil
- Immobilize the patient using sponges and straps

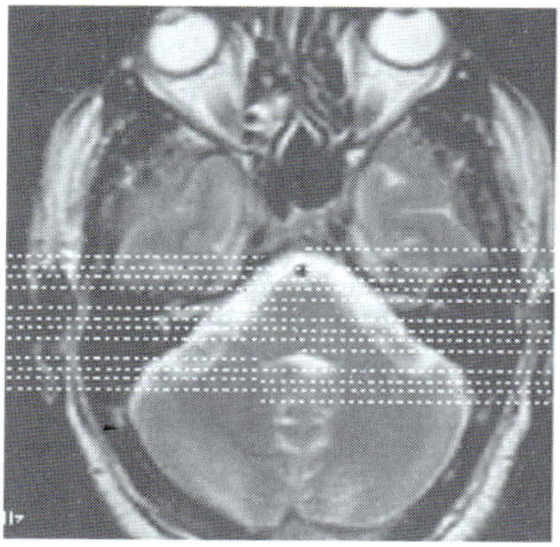

Axial localizer for coronal slices

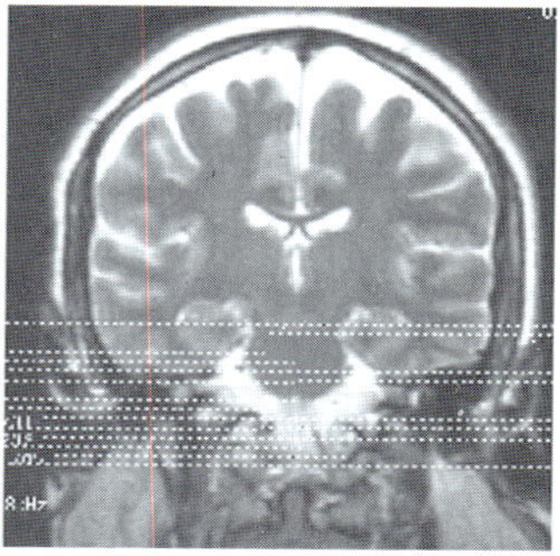

Coronal localizer for axial slices

PROTOCOL: POSTERIOR FOSSA AND INTERNAL AUDITORY MEATUS

Indication

- Symptoms that require the exclusion of an acoustic neuroma (vertigo, unilateral sensory hearing loss, tinnitus)
- Facial palsy / numbness, • Diagnosis of a posterior fossa lesion
- Hemifacial spasm, • Trigeminal neuralgia

Sequences

Pulse Sequence	Axial T2	Axial T1	*Axial T1+C-FS	COR T1	Axial 3DT2	AX-T1 FS-FSE
TR	4000	450	600	650	4000	450
TE/IR	85	Min	Min	Min	130	Min
ETL	20	—	—	2	64	2
Bandwidth	15.63	15.63	15.63	20.83	15.63	20.83
Nex	5	3	2	4	1	4
Slice	3	3	3	3	0.8	3
Gap	0	0	0	0	LOCS per slab;30	0
No. of Slices	12	12	12	11	No. of slab 1	12
Matrix Freq/Phase	320/256	256/256	256/224	320/256	256/256	320/256
FOV	18	18	18	18	18	18
SNR	100	100	100	100	100	100
Scan Time	4.37	5.45	4.32	5.30	8.01	7.34
Frequency Direction	R/L	R/L	A/P	S/I	R/L	R/L
Auto Center Frequency	Water	Water	Water	Water	Water	Water
Flow Compensation Direction	Slice	—	—	—	Slice	Slice
Saturation	A,P,S,I	S,I	S,I FAT	S,I	A,P,S,I	S,I FAT

Contrast Usage: Inject Gadolinium (10 ml) if pathological condition seen. Acquire post-contrast T1W images in all 3 planes

PITUITARY

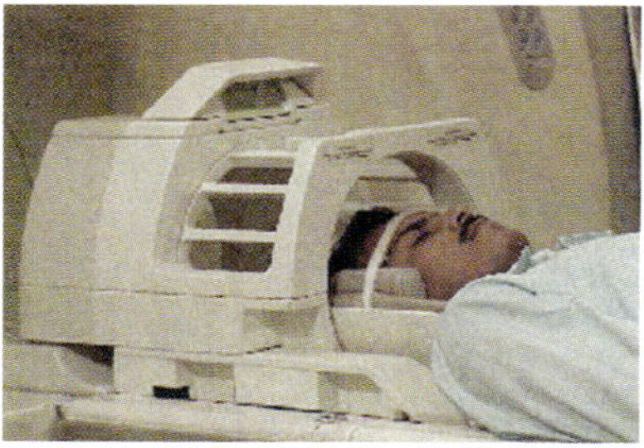

Patient Position-Head Coil

Patient Position-Head coil:
- Set-up the head coil
- Place the patient in the head coil
- Immobilize the patient using sponges and straps

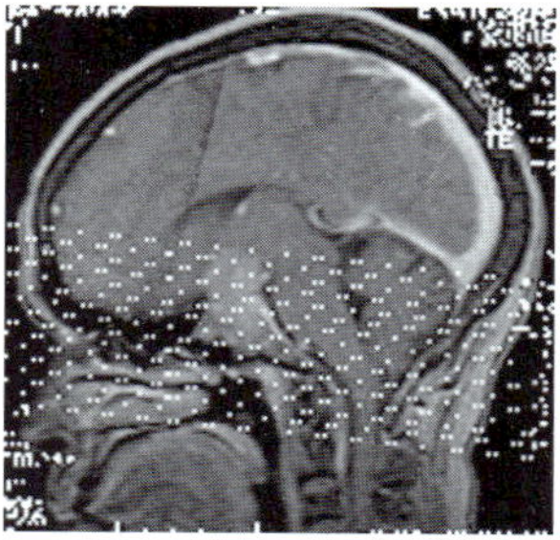

Sagittal localizer for axial slices

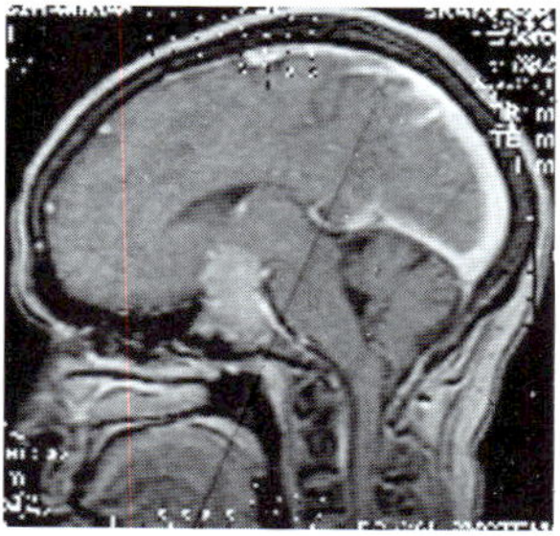

Sagittal localizer for coronal slices

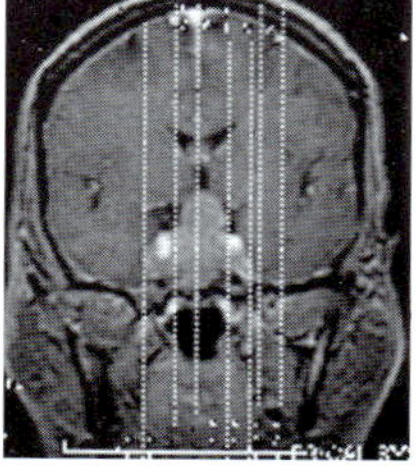

Coronal localizer for sagittal slices

PROTOCOL: PITUITARY

Indication

Investigation of diseases related to pituitary function (hyperprolactinaemia, Cunhing's disease, acromegaly, hypopituitarism, diabetes insipidus, amenorrhea)

• Hypothalamic disorders, • Visual field defect, • Pre- and postoperative assessment of pituitary adenomas

Sequences

Pulse Sequence	AxialT2	COR T1	COR T2	Sag T1	Sag T1+C-fs	Cor T1+C-dyn-FSE
TR	4900	450	4000	450	650	400
TE/IR	85	Min	85	Min	Min-full	Min
ETL	16	—	24	—	—	4
Bandwidth	20.83	10.42	20.83	10.42	12.50	20.83
Nex	2	3	4	3	3	1
Slice	5	3	3	3	3	3
Gap	1.5	0.3	0.3	0.3	0.3	0
No. of Slices	20	11	12	11	12	6
Matrix Freq/Phase	256/256	256/192	256/256	256/192	256/192	256/160
FOV/Phase FOV	24/ .75	18	18	18	18	20/ .75
SNR	100	100	100	100	100	100
Scan Time	2.02	4.20	3.20	4.20	6.17	0.14
Frequency Direction	A/P	S/I	S/I	S/I	S/I	S/I
Auto Center Frequency	Water	Water	Water	Water	Water	Water
Flow Compensation Direction	Slice	—	Freq	—	—	—
Saturation	I	I	I	I	I,FAT	S,I

Contrast Usage: Inject Gadolinium (10 ml), if pathological condition seen

Remarks: Dynamic scans should be taken after IV contrast/Coronal images should be taken first/Acquire postcontrast T1W images in all 3 planes

ORBITS

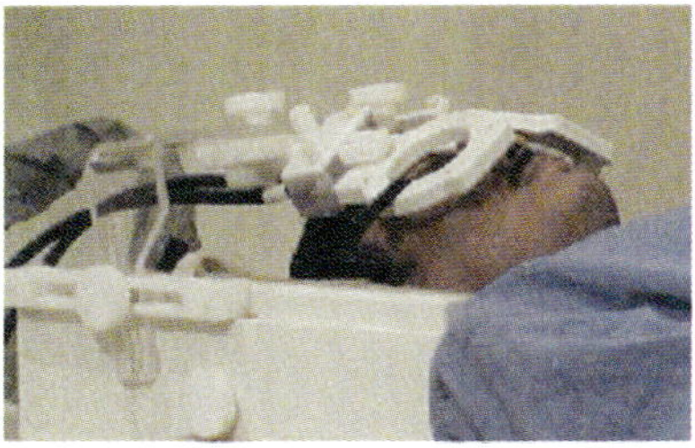

Patient Position-Surface Coils

- Before you bring the patient into the scan room, have the patient remove all eye make-up.
- Position the patient supine with the head in the positioner.
- Place the chin up with the Orbital-meatal line +15 to the table top. This position places the optic nerve perpendicular to the table
- Turn on the alignment lights. Place the sagittal light on the mid-sagittal line of the patient's head and the axial line to pass through both outer canthus of the eyes.
- Place the coils parallel to the anatomy and as close as possible to the eye without touching the patient.
- Immobilize the patient using sponges and straps

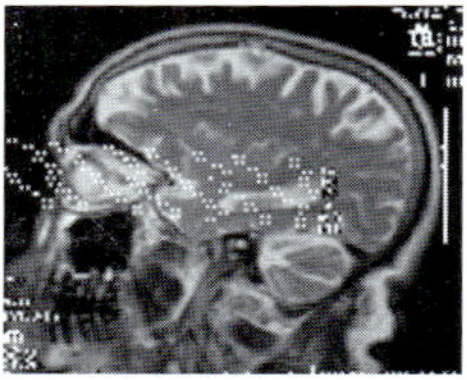

Sagittal image of the orbit and optic nerve showing the correct placement of axial oblique slices parallel to the optic nerve

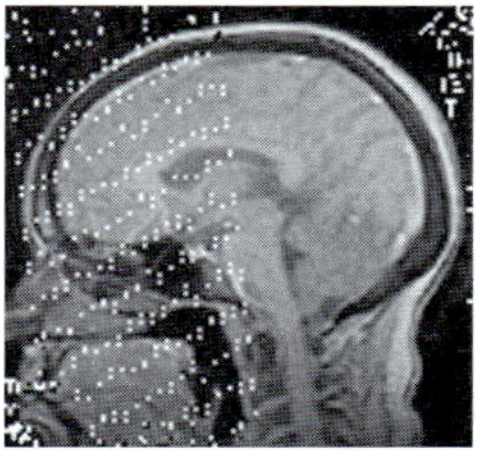

Sagittal image showing correct placement of coronal slices

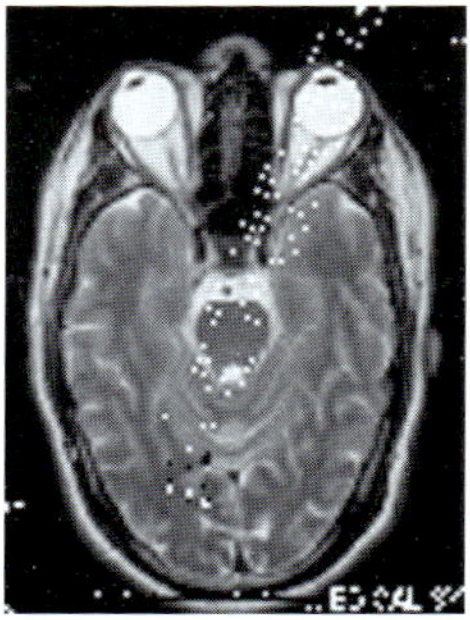

Axial oblique image of the orbits clearly demonstrating the lens of eye, the globe, the optic nerves and the optic chiasma

PROTOCOL: ORBITS

Indication:

- Visual disturbance
- Proptosis
- Evaluation of orbital or ocular mass lesions

Sequences

Pulse Sequence	Ax T2	Ax T1	COR T2	Sag T1	Sag T2-fs	Sag FATSAT T1
TR	4000	450	4000	400	4050	400
TE/IR	85	Min full	85	Min	85	Min
ETL	16	——	16	——	24	——
Bandwidth	20.83	15.63	12.50	15.63	20.83	15.63
Nex	2	2	4.00	2.00	3	2
Slice	5	3	3	3	3	3
Gap	1.5	0	0	0	0	0
No. of Slices	20	12	1	12	12	12
Matrix Freq/Phase	256/256	256/224	256/224	256/224	256/192	256/224
FOV	24	16	16	16	16	16
SNR	115	100	55	100	100	100
Scan Time	2.16	3.20	3.52	3.02	1.41	6.04
Frequency						
Direction	A/P	A/P	S/I	R/L	S/I	S/I
Auto Center Frequency	Water	Water	Water	Water	Water	Water
Flow Compensation Direction	Slice	——	Freq	——	Freq	——
Saturation	I	S,I	——	S,I	S,I FAT	S,I FAT

Contrast Usage: Inject Gadolinium(10 ml) ,if pathological conditions seen. Acquire post-contrast TI WI images in all 3 planes

TEMPOROMANDIBULAR JOINT

Patient Position- dual 3 inch Coil

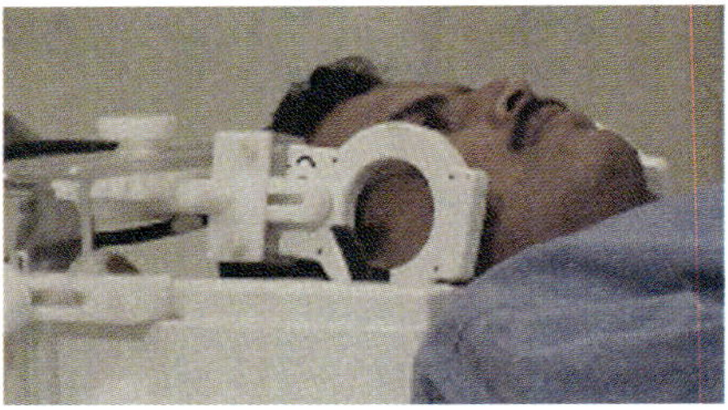

Closed Mouth

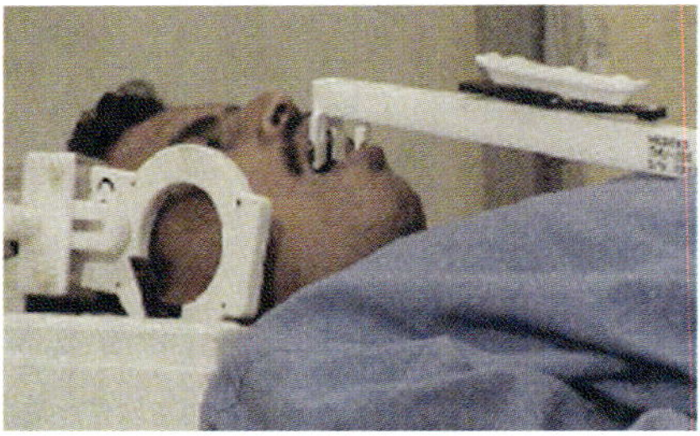

Open Mouth (Mouth Opening Device)

Patient Position-dual 3 inch coil

perform both closed and open mouth sagittal views

R 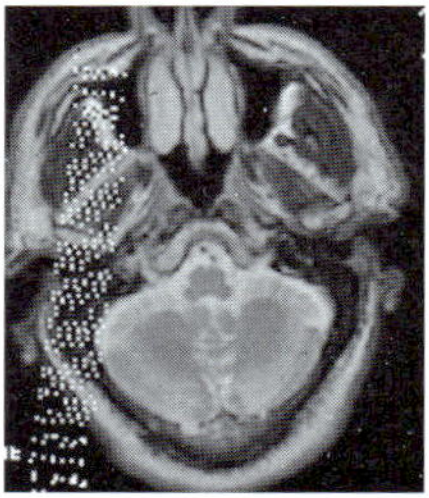 L

Right TM Joint

R 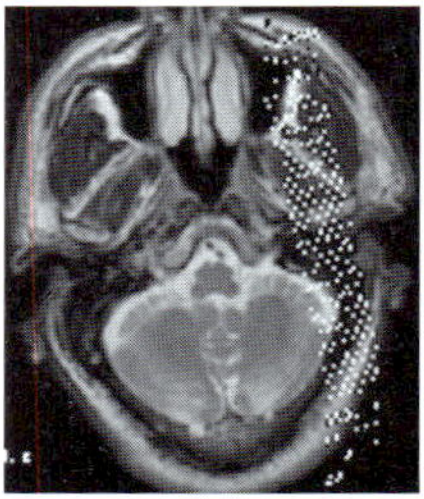 L

Left TM Joint

Axial localizer through the TM joint showing correct placement of sagittal oblique slices perpendicular to the Mandibular Condyles

PROTOCOL: TEMPOROMANDIBULAR JOINT

Indication

- Suspected internal meniscal derangement

Sequences

Pulse Sequence	Sag T1 FSE	Sag T2 FSE	Sag T2* GRE	CorT2* GRE	Cor T1 SE	Sag 3D T2*GRE
TR	450	2600	300	350	400	29.0
TE/IR	Min	85	15.0	15	Min	12.0
ETL	3	16	FA-20Deg	FA-20Deg	—	FA-20Deg
Bandwidth	20.83	20.83	8.93	8.93	8.93	8.93
Nex	4	4	3	3	3	2
Slice	2	2	2	2	2	1.2
Gap	0	0	0	0	0	Overlap locs;2
No. of Slices	9	9	11	11	12	Locs per slab:24
Matrix Freq/Phase	256/224	256/224	256/192	256/192	256/192	256/128
FOV	12	12	12	16	16	12
SNR	100	100	100	100	100	100
Scan Time	2.13	2.31	2.56	3.19	3.56	3.01
Frequency Direction	S/I	S/I	S/I	S/I	S/I	S/I
Auto Center Frequency	Water	Water	Water	Water	Water	Water
Flow Compensation Direction	—	—	—	—	—	—
Saturation	—	—	—	—	—	—

Remarks: Inject Gadolinium (10 ml), if pathological conditions seen acquire post-contrast T1 WI images in all 3 planes

DIFFUSION

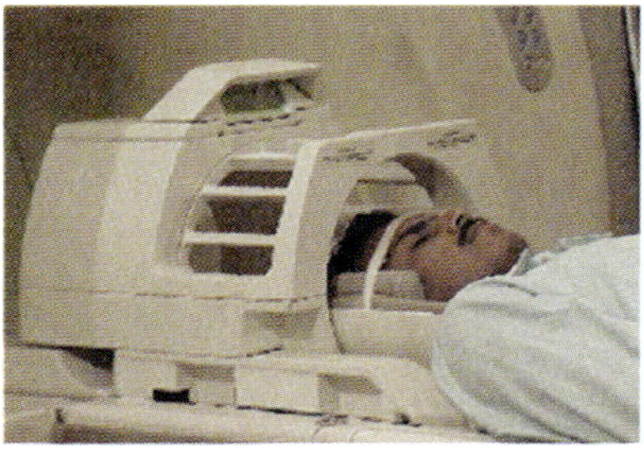

Patient Position-Head Coil

Patient Position-Head coil:
- Set-up the head coil
- Place the patient in the head coil
- Immobilize the patient using sponges and straps

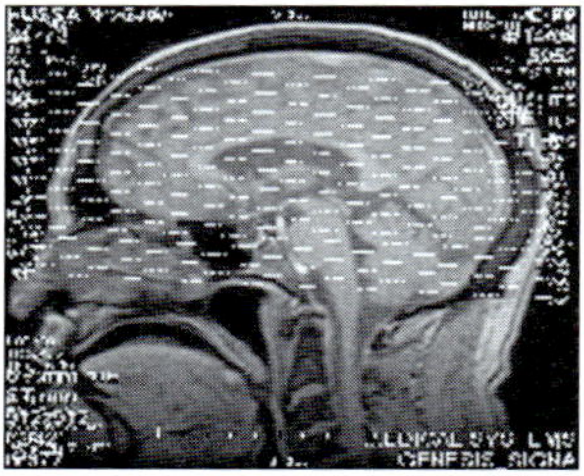

Sagittal localizer for axial slices

PROTOCOL: DIFFUSION

Indication

- Early detection of cerebral infarction
- Differentiating between arachnoid cysts versus epidermoid
- To differentiate cerebral abscess from necrotic tumor
- In the evaluation of patients with multiple sclerosis

Sequences

Pulse Sequence	O-Axial T2 DW-EPI	O-Axial FLAIR DW-EPI
TR	10,000	10,000
TE/IR	Minimum	Minimum
ETL	—	Inv.Time:2500
Bandwidth	—	—
Nex	1	1.00
Slice	5	5
Gap	0	0
No. of Slices	25	25
Matrix Freq/Phase	96/128	128/128
FOV/Phase FOV	36/0.60	36/0.60
SNR	100	100
Scan Time	0.40	2.00
Frequency Direction	A/P	R/L
Auto Center Frequency	Water	Water
Flow Compensation Direction	—	—
Saturation	I	—

Remarks: B-Value 1000

Diffusion direction: ALL

PERFUSION

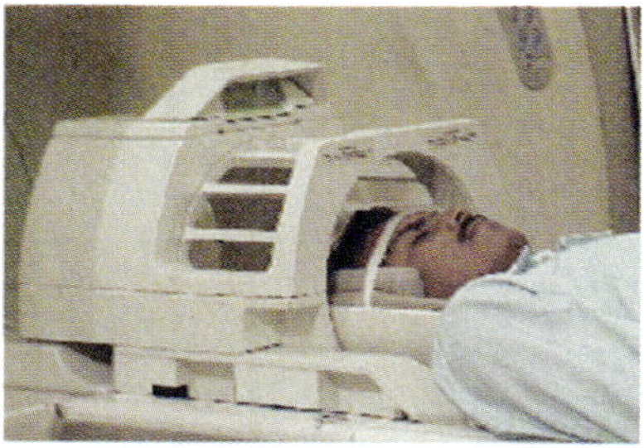

Patient Position-Head Coil

Patient Position-Head coil:
- Set-up the head coil
- Place the patient in the head coil
- Immobilize the patient using sponges and straps

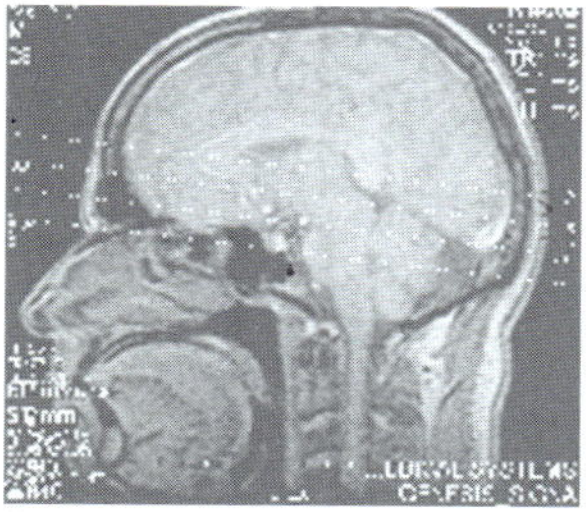

Sagittal localizer for axial slices

PROTOCOL: PERFUSION

Indication

- For the evaluation of hyper acute stroke
- For the evaluation of brain tumors (for tumor grading, sterotactic biopsy guidance, distinguishing radiation necrosis from recurrent glioma and determining prognosis and response to treatment)
- For the evaluation of epilepsy and Alzheimer's type dementia.

Sequences

Pulse Sequence	No. of Shots O-Ax dyn EPI SE-EPI
TR	2000
TE/IR	60
ETL	FA-90 Degrees
Bandwidth	62.50
Nex	1
Slice	10
Gap	0
No. of Slices	12
Matrix	
Freq/Phase	96/64
FOV	30
SNR	100
Scan Time	1.20
Frequency Direction	R/L
Auto Center Frequency	Water
Flow Compensation Direction	—
Saturation	—

Contrast Usage: Contrast -20 ml

Remarks: All image data has to be transferred to work station for further evaluation.

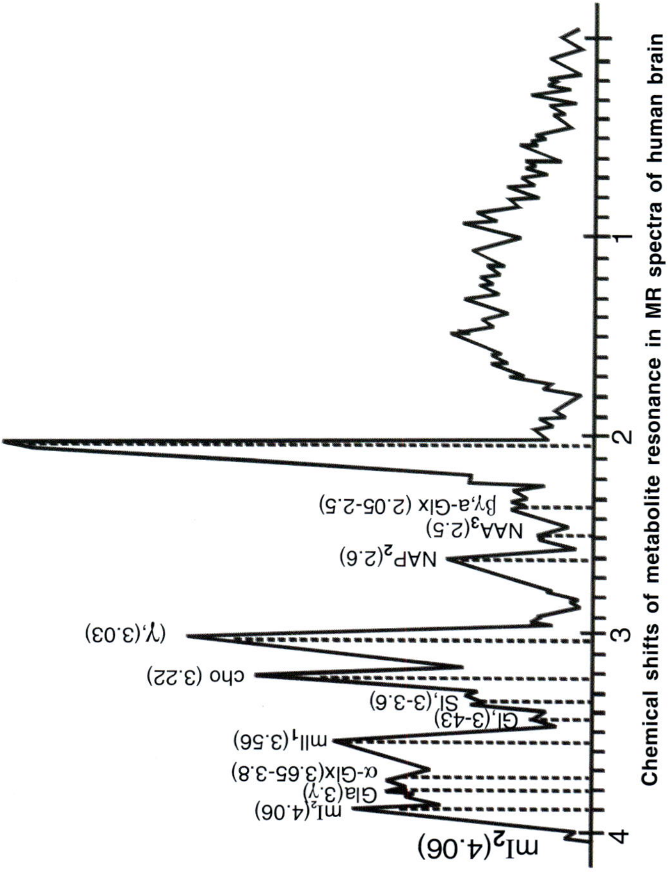
Chemical shifts of metabolite resonance in MR spectra of human brain
4
3
2
1
cho (3.22)

N-acetylaspartate (first peak, NAA_1)	2.02
β-γ-Glutamine and glutamate (β, γ-Glx)	2.05-2.5
N-acetylaspartate (second peak, NAA_2)	2.6
N-acetylaspartate (third peak, NAA_3)	2.5
Total creatine (Cr)	3.03
Total choline (Cho)	3.22
Scyllo-inositol (SI)	3.30
Glucose	3.43
Myo-inositol (ml)	3.5
α-Glutamine and Glutamate (α-Glx)	3.65
Second peak of glucose	3.8
Second peak of Cr	3.9
Second peak of ml	4.06

SPECTROSCOPY

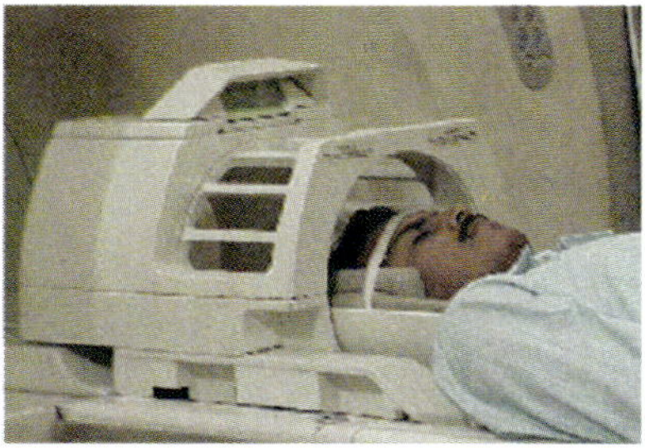

Patient Position-Head Coil

Patient Position-Head coil:

- Set-up the head coil
- Place the patient in the head coil
- Immobilize the patient using sponges and straps

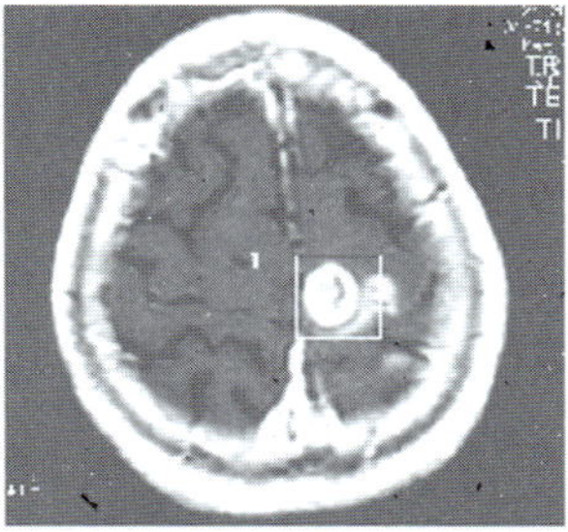

Axial localizer for spectroscopy

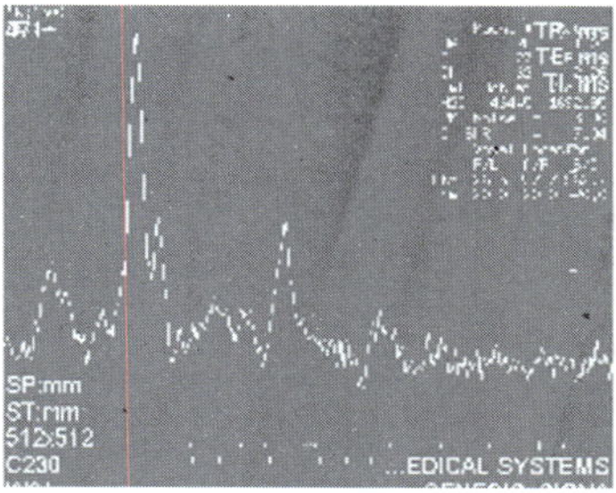

Spectroscopic image

PROTOCOL: SPECTROSCOPY

Indication

- In the evaluation of brain tumors,
- Radiation injury,
- For the evaluation of hyper acute stroke,
- In cases of mesial temporal sclerosis
- In the evaluation of pediatric degenerative and metabolic disorders,
- Alzheimer's disease,
- To differentiate pyogenic abscesses from brain tumors

Sequences

Pulse Sequence	Localizer for Spectroscopy	Ax probe SV-Press 35 TE	Ax probe SV-Press 144TE	Ax probe SV-Press 288TE	AX-Probe-SV-STEAM 30TE	Multi voxel Axial Probe SI Press-144TE
TR	3000	1500	1500	1500	2000	1000
TE/IR	85.0	35.0	144	288	30.0	144.0
ETL	24	—		—	—	—
Bandwidth	20.83	—		—	—	—
Nex	0.50	8	8	8	8	1.00
Slice/Voxel Thickness	20	20	20	20	20	10
Gap	0		—	—	—	—
No. of Slices	9	1	1	1	1	1
Matrix Freq/Phase	256/192	1/1	1/1	1/1	—	16/16
FOV	24	24	24	24	24	24
SNR	100	100	100	100	100	100
Scan Time	0.24	2.12	3.48	3.48	5.04	4.20
Frequency Direction	A/P	A/P	A/P	A/P	A/P	A/P
Auto Center Frequency	Water	Water	Water	Water	Water	Water
Flow Compensation Direction	Slice	—	—	—	—	—
Saturation	—	—	—	—	—	—

Remarks: The study takes approximately six minutes and can be add-on to a routine brain MRI. MRS provides a brain map of chemical spectra and biochemical information about the tissues.

FUNCTIONAL

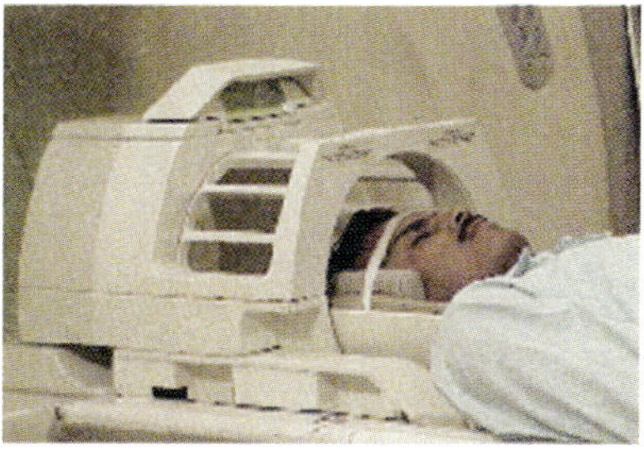

Patient Position-Head coil:

- Set-up the head coil
- Place the patient in the head coil
- Immobilize the patient using sponges and straps

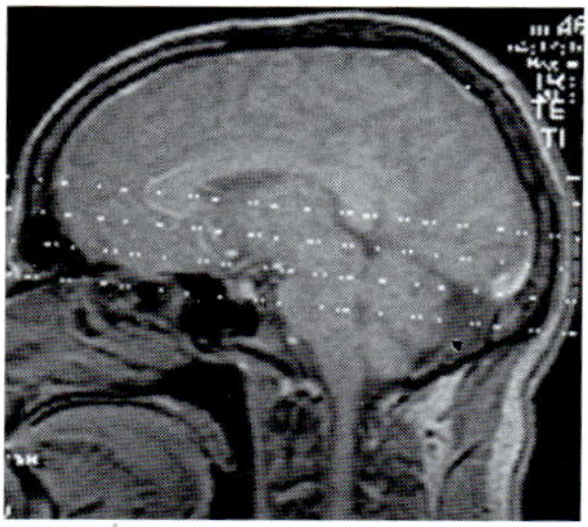

Sagittal localizer for axial slices

PROTOCOL: FUNCTIONAL

Indication:

- To map sensorimotor functions in patients with a variety of brain pathology such as tumors, arteriovenous and cavernous malformations and cortical dysplasias
- For the detection of language areas
- To map primary auditory cortex and visual cortex

Sequences

Pulse Sequence	O-Axial tc-EPI GR-EPI 4 locs	Axial SE:T1
TR	3000	440
TE/IR	60	15
ETL	Flip Angle:90 Deg	—
Bandwidth	62.50	15.6
Nex	1.00	2
Slice	10	10
Gap	2	0
No. of Slices	4	4
Matrix		
Freq/Phase	64/64	256/224
FOV	40	40
SNR	100	100
Scan Time	6.26	3.20
Frequency Direction	R/L	A/P
Auto Center Frequency	Water	Water
Flow Compensation Direction	—	—
Saturation	—	—

Remarks: Functional imaging maps out specific regions of brain corresponding to various functions such as motor, sensory, visual and language. This technique has an important role to play in patients with neoplasms opting for surgery, as well as psychiatric disorders.

MRA-HEAD

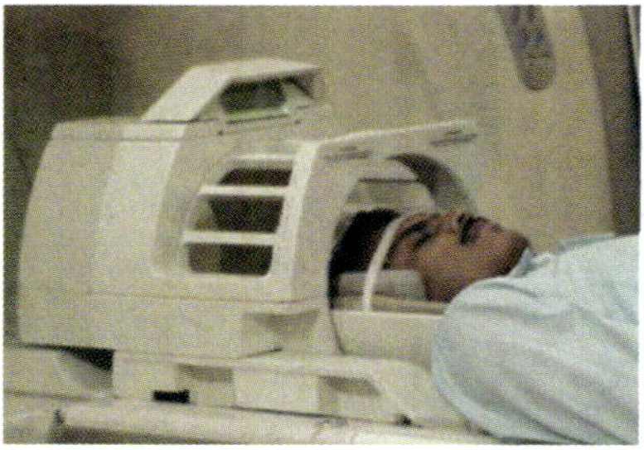

Patient Position-Head Coil

Patient Position-Head coil:
- Set-up the head coil
- Place the patient in the head coil
- Immobilize the patient using sponges and straps

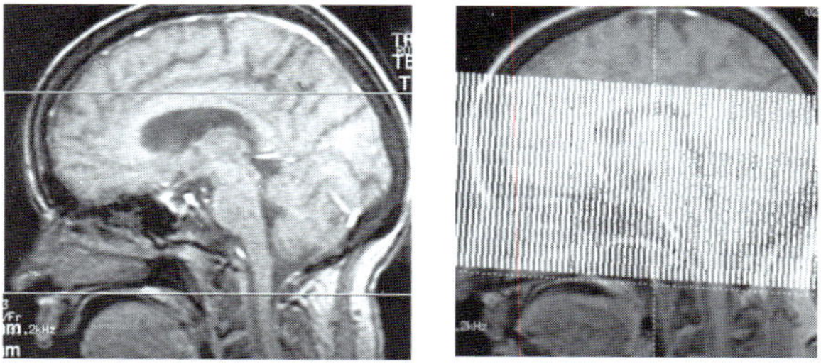

MRA 3D TOF single slab

PROTOCOL: MRA-HEAD

Indication

- Circle of Willis (stroke or TIA)

Sequences

Pulse Sequence	AX 3D TOF: 1 slab	AX3D TOF:4 slab
TR	36	36
TE	6.9	6.9
Flip Angle	20 Deg.	20 Deg.
Bandwidth	15.63	15.63
Nex	1	1
Slice Thickness	1.2	1.2
Overlap Locations	12	2
Locations per slab	64	20
Matrix		
Freq/Phase	256/192	256/192
FOV	20	20
SNR	100	100
Scan Time	7.25	7.05
Frequency Direction	A/P	A/P
Auto Center Frequency	Water	Water
Flow Compensation Direction	—	—
Saturation	S	S

MRV

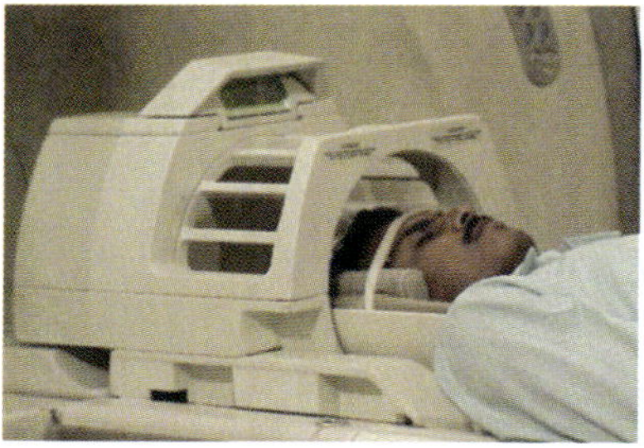

Patient Position-Head coil:

- Set-up the head coil
- Place the patient in the head coil
- Immobilize the patient using sponges and straps

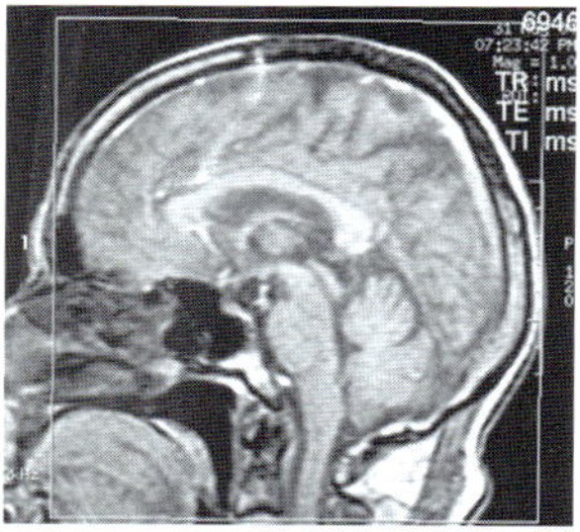

MRV 2D TOF

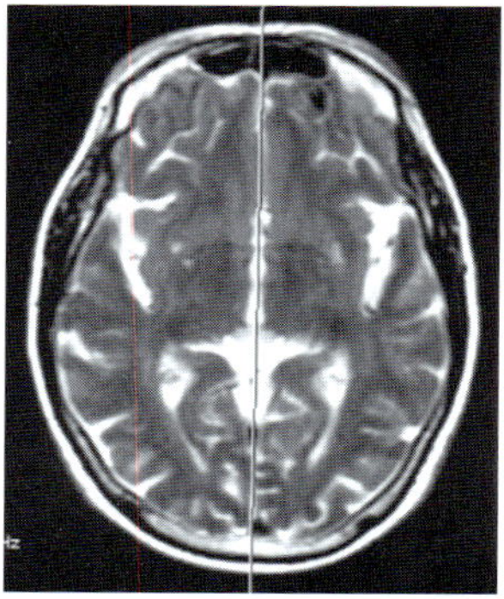

MRV 2D -PC (Sagittal)

Protocol: MRV-Head

Indication

- Deep venous and superficial sinus thrombosis

Sequences

Pulse Sequence	Sag 2D PC	Cor 2D PC	Axial PC	Cor 2D TOF
TR	33	33	33.0	Minimum
TE/IR	—	—	—	Minimum
Flip Angle	20 Deg.	20 Deg.	20 Deg.	15 Deg.
Bandwidth	—	—	—	15.63
Nex	4	4	4.00	1.00
Slice Thickness	40	40	15.0	1.5
Gap	0	0	0	—
No. of Slices	1	1	5	120
Matrix Freq/Phase	256/256	256/256	256/160	256/128
FOV	24	24	22	22
SNR	100	100	100	100
Scan Time	2.15	2.15	5.19	4.54
Frequency Direction	S/I	S/I	A/P	S/I
Auto Center Frequency	Water	Water	Water	Water
Flow Compensation Direction	—	—	—	—
Saturation	—	—	—	Inferior
Velocity Encoding	15.0	15.0	60.0	

STERIOTACTIC BIOPSY PROCEDURE

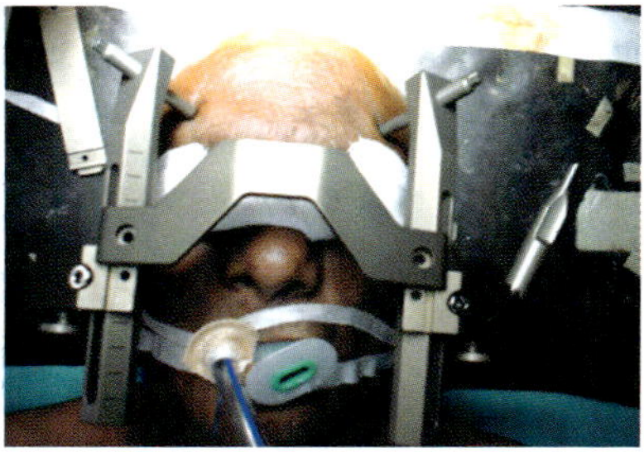

Patient with Steriotactic Frame

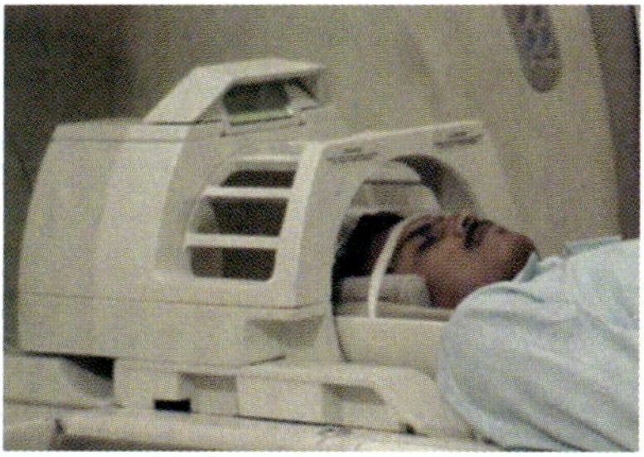

Patient Position-Head coil

Patient Position-Head coil:

- Set-up the head coil
- Place the patient in the head coil with stereotactic frame
- Immobilize the patient using sponges and straps

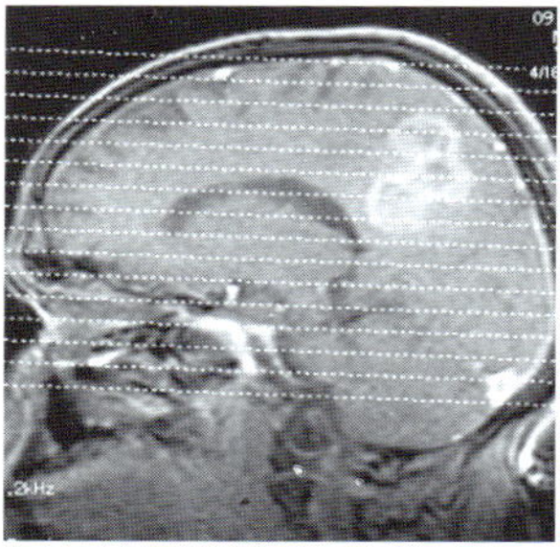

Sagittal localizer for axial slices for biopsy site

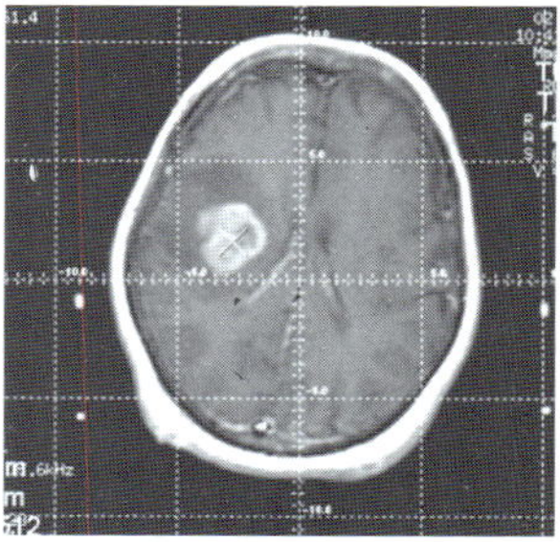

Post-contrast T1W axial image

PROTOCOL: STEREOTACTIC BIOPSY

Indication

- Deep seated , small, eloquent-location of the lesion
- Diagnosis in doubt?
- When lesions are multiple and small

Sequences

Pulse Sequence	AX SET1 Post-contrast	AX SE T1 Post BX
TR	400	400
TE/IR	9.0	9.0
ETL	—	—
Bandwidth	15.83	15.83
Nex	2	2
Slice	6	6
Gap	1.5	1.5
No. of Slices	16	16
Matrix Freq/Phase	256/192	256/192
FOV	26	26
SNR	105	105
Scan Time	2.40	2.40
Frequency Direction	A/P	A/P
Auto Center Frequency	Water	Water
Flow Compensation Direction	—	—
Saturation	I	I

Remarks:

- MR Compatible Stereotactic frame is fixed to the patients head by a surgeon.
- The biopsy site will be selected on post-contrast T1W axial image
- Post-procedure plain axial T1W image should be taken to know weather biopsy was taken from the target side or not
- To see any postoperative hematoma formation or injury to the eloquent areas

DEEP BRAIN STIMULATION(DBS)

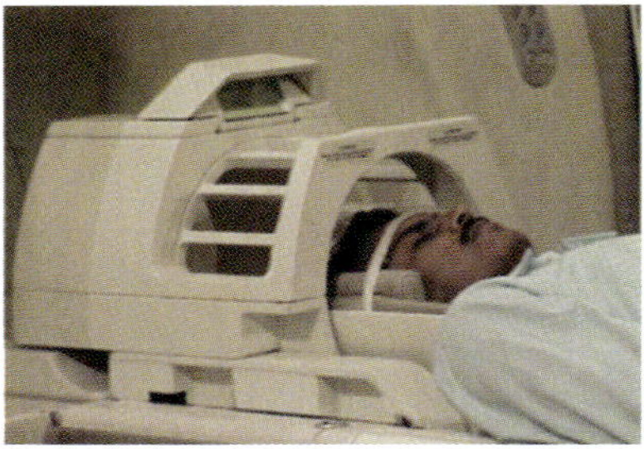

Patient Position-Head coil:

- Set-up the head coil
- Place the patient in the head coil with stereotaxy frame
- Immobilize the patient using sponges and straps

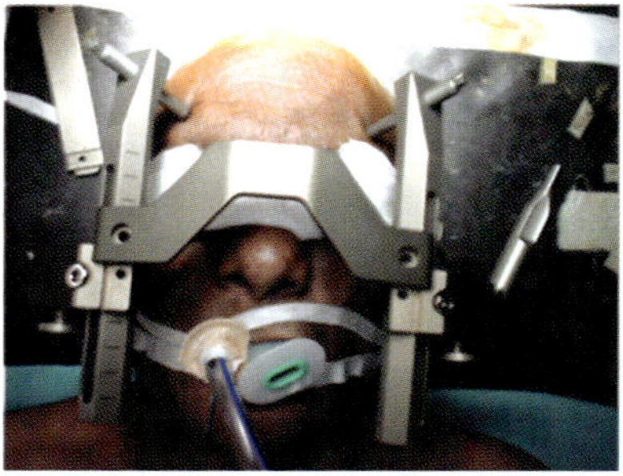

Patient fixed with stereotaxy frame

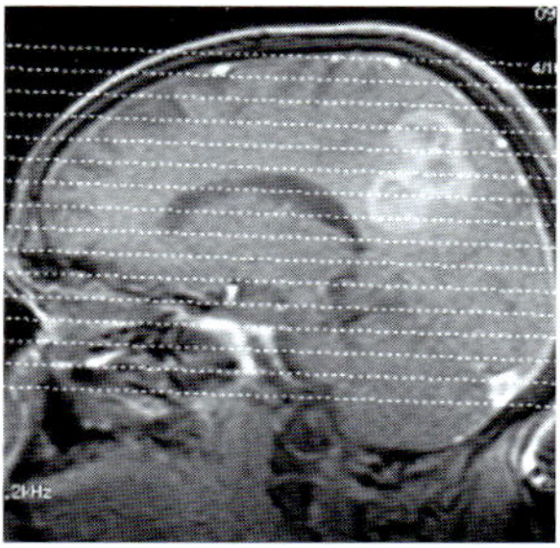

Sagittal localizer for axial slices

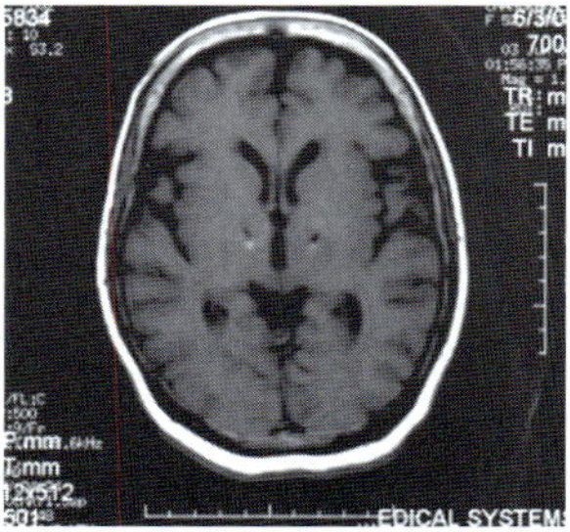

Post DBS T1 W axial

PROTOCOL: D.B.S (DEEP BRAIN STIMULATION)

Indication:

Identification of Anterior Commisure, Posterior Commisure, Sub-thalamic nucleus, palladium and thalamic nuclei

Usually done for movement disorder (i.e., Parkinson's disease, essential tremor, dystonia)

Sequences

Pulse Sequence	Sag T1 SE	Axial T1 SE	Cor T2 SE	Axial T1 FSE (Post DBS)
TR	500	500	2500	525
TE/IR	10	10	90	Min
ETL	—	—	—	2
Bandwidth	15.63	20.83	15.63	20.83
Nex	2	2	1	1
Slice	3	2	3	5
Gap	1	1	0	1.5
No. of Slices	16	16	16	20
Matrix Freq/Phase	256/256	256/192	256/192	256/256
FOV	26	26	26	24
SNR	103	105	112	100
Scan Time	4.20	3.16	16.10	1.44
Frequency Direction	S/I	A/P	S/I	A/P
Auto Center Frequency	Water	Water	Water	Water
Flow Compensation Direction	—	—	—	—
Saturation	I	I	I	I

Remarks: -Obtain Post-procedure axial and coronal T1W images to see the correct position of the electrodes and to detect any complication.

CSF FLOW

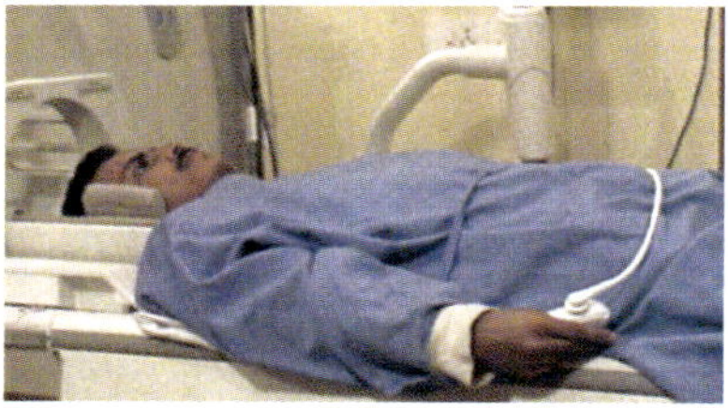

Patient Position-Head Coil with Peripheral Gating

- Set-up the head coil
- Place the patient in the head coil
- Immobilize the patient using sponges and straps

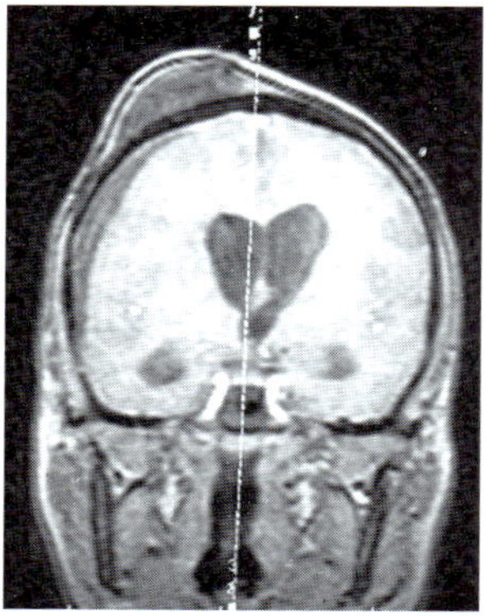

Coronal localizer for sagittal slices

PROTOCOL: CSF-FLOW

Indication

- For the evaluation of normal pressure hydrocephalus (NPH)
- Evaluation of third ventriculostomy
- Evaluation of intracranial cystic or other cisternal lesions
- Evaluation of chiari 1 malformation
- Evaluation of spinal canal

  (Causes of syringomyelia like arachnoiditis, intradural scarring, arachnoid cysts)

Sequences

Pulse Sequence	O-Sag Cine PC CSF Flow	Quantitative flow analysis	Axial T2 FSE
TR	33.0	40	4900
TE/IR	—	—	85
ETL	FA:20 Deg	FA:15 Deg	16
Bandwidth	—	—	20.83
Nex	2.00	1.00	2
Slice	5.00	4.00	5
Gap	0	0	1.5
No. of Slices	1	1	20
Matrix Freq/Phase	256/192	256/256	256 / 256
FOV	24	16	24
SNR	100	100	100
Scan Time	3.54	2.35	2.02
Frequency Direction	S/I	A/P	A/P
Auto Center Frequency	Water	Water	Water
Flow Compensation Direction	—	—	Slice
Saturation	——	——	I

Remarks:

I. Retrospectively cardiac gate to 32 cine phase

II. Angle perpendicular to aqueduct (for R/O Shunt malfunction: venc=2 cm/sec)

III. Peripheral gating

PROTOCOL: CSF-RHINORRHOEA/OTORRHOEA

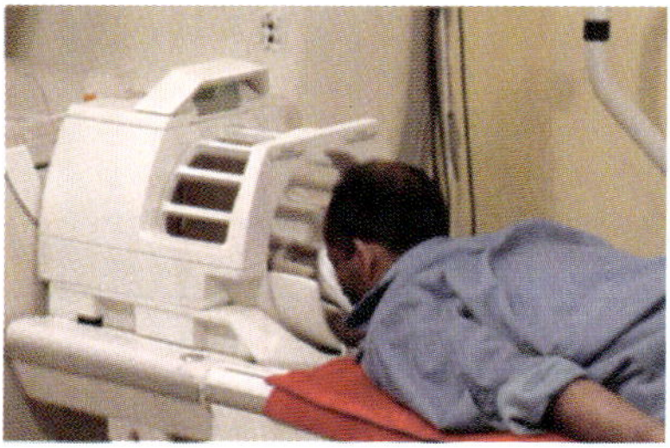

Patient Position- Prone

Patient Position-Head coil:

- Set-up the head coil
- Place the patient prone in the head coil
- Immobilize the patient using sponges and straps

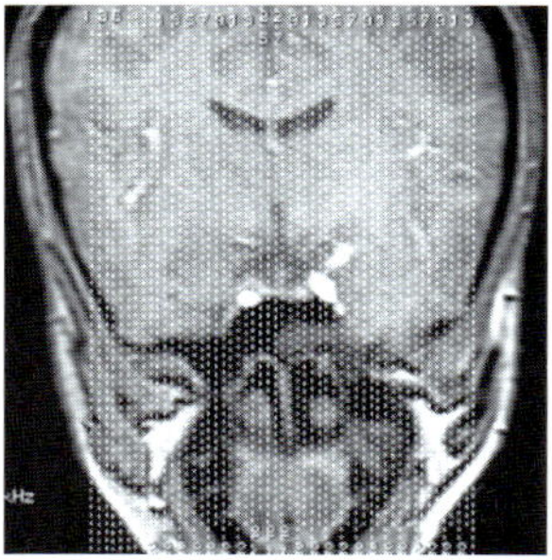

Coronal localizer for sagittal slices

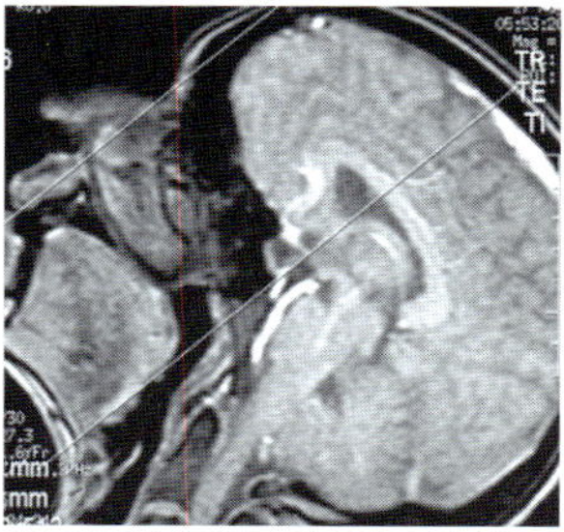

Sagittal localizer to obtain coronal images

(Patient prone)

PROTOCOL: CSF-RHINORRHOEA/OTORRHOEA

Indication

Post-traumatic watery discharge from nose and ears

Sequences

Pulse Sequence	Heavily WI Cor-T2	Heavily WI Sag-T2	Heavily WI Axial-T2
TR	6000	6000	6000
TE/IR	250	250	250
ETL	20	20	20
Bandwidth	15.63	15.63	15.63
Nex	3	3	3
Slice	2	2	2
Gap	Interleave	Interleave	Interleave
No. of Slices	40	40	40
Matrix Freq/Phase	256/256	256/256	256/256
FOV	30	30	30
SNR	100	100	100
Scan Time	6.12	6.12	6.12
Frequency Direction	S/I	S/I	S/I
Auto Center Frequency	Water	Water	Water
Flow Compensation Direction	Frequency	Frequency	Frequency
Saturation			

MRA-NECK

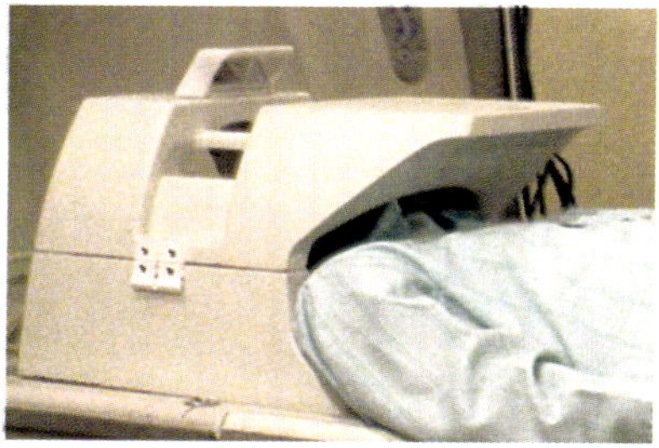

Patient Position-Vascular Neck

Patient Position:

- Position the patient supine, head first .use sponges or the head holder to support the patient's head. Elevate the head slightly for the best coil fit.
- Place the coil to cover the head and neck.
- Turn on the alignment lights and center the patient's midline (nose and sternal notch) to the sagittal light.
- Move the coil as close to the patient's jaw as possible.
- Use sponges or cushions as needed for patient comfort.
- Landmark at the centre of the coil.
- Instruct the patient to breath evenly and minimize swallowing.

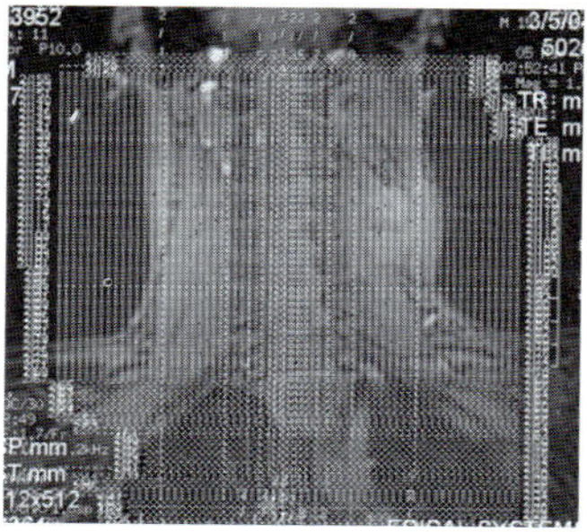

Coronal localizer for axial slices

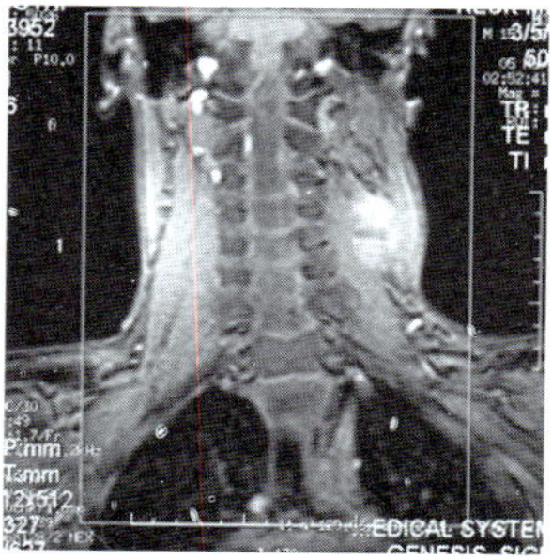

Axial slab to obtain axial slices

PROTOCOL: MRA-NECK

Indication:

- Cervical Carotid Arteries-T1A 'S, Strokes, Dissections, Occlusions

Sequences

Pulse Sequence	AX 2D TOF SPGR, pg	AX 3D TOF 6 Slabs	Coronal vasc. TOF SPGR
TR	Minimum	26.0	—
TE	Minimum	6.9	Minimum
ETL/Flip Angle	FA-45 Deg.	20	FA-45 Deg.
Bandwidth	31.25	15.63	31.25
Nex	1.00	1.00	1.00
Slice	2.0	2.4	1.4
Gap/Overlap Locations	0	5/20	No. of Slabs:1
No. of Slices/Slabs	101	6	Locations per slab:44
Matrix Freq/Phase	256/160	256/128	256/224
FOV	20	20	24
SNR	100	100	100
Scan Time	20.14	5.45	0.49
Frequency Direction	R/L	R/L	S/I
Auto Center Frequency	Water	Water	Water
Flow Compensation Direction	—	—	—
Saturation	S	S	—
			> Smart Prep. >Contrast

Remarks: Peripheral Gating

SPINE

CERVICAL SPINE

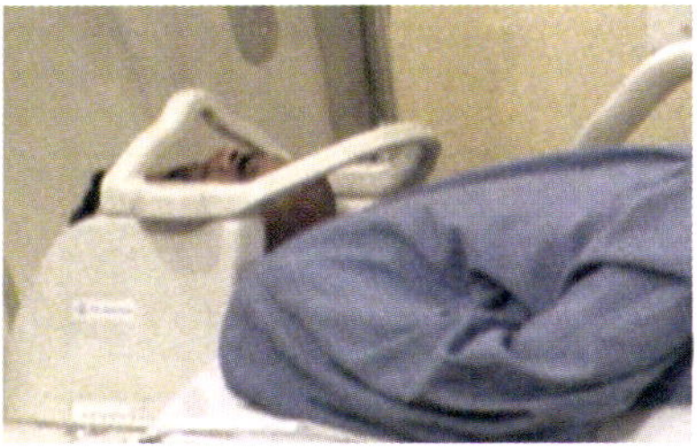

Patient position-CTL-Top

Patient Position:

- Place the coil on the magnet table and plug it in
- Place patient supine, head first. Rest the head and neck in the coil
- Position the superior end of the coil at the base of the skull. This position should include C1 on a sagittal image so that you can count vertebra for localization purpose.

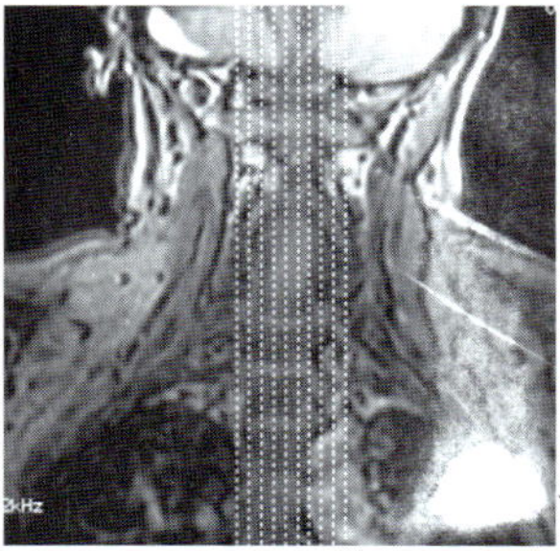

Coronal localizer for sagittal slices

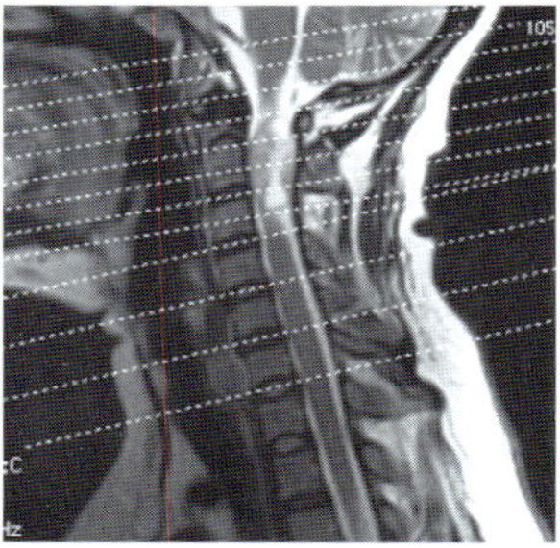

Sagittal C-spine showing axial-oblique slice positions parallel to each disc spaces

PROTOCOL: CERVICAL SPINE

Indication

- Cervical myelopathy
- Cervical cord compression or trauma
- Assessment of extent of spinal infection or tumor
- Diagnosis of chiari malformation and cervical syrinx (total extent of syrinx must be determined. Whole spine imaging may be necessary).
- Visualization of MS plaques within the cord.

Sequences

Pulse Sequence	Sag T2	Sag T1	Sag ST1R	Axial T2	Axial T1	Cor T1
TR	3000	475	2700	3000	500	575
TE/IR	102	15	50/150	102	Min	13
ETL	18	2	6	16	2	2
Band width	31.25	13.89	15.63	31.25	11.36	20.83
Nex	4	3	2	4	3	2
Slice	3	3	3	4	4	3
Gap	1	1	1	3	3	1
No. of slices	11	11	11	11	11	9
Matrix Freq/Phase	256/192	256/192	256/192	256/192	256/192	320/256
FOV	24	24	24	22	22	26
SNR	100	100	85	100	100	100
Scan Time	2.18	2.14	2.58	2.30	2.26	2.25
Frequency Direction	A/P	S/I	A/P	A/P	A/P	S/I
Auto Center Frequency	Water	Water	Water	Water	Water	Water
Flow Compensation Direction	——	——	Slice	Slice	——	——
Saturation	——	——	——	——	——	a

THORACIC SPINE

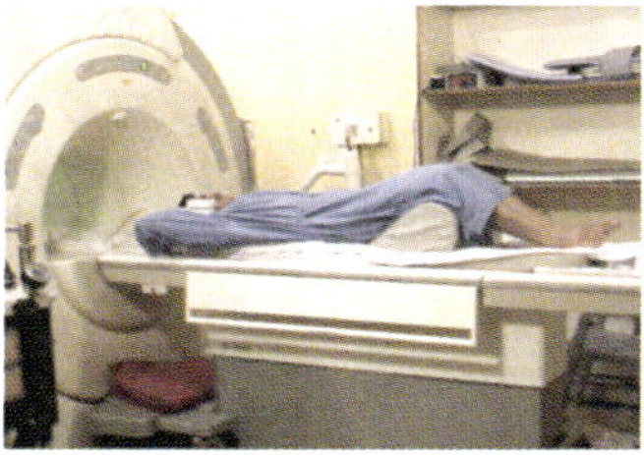

Patient Position-Phased Array Coil-CTL Mid

- Place the phased array coil on the magnet table and plug the phased array coil port.
- Position patient supine, and either head or feet first. A feet first position may be preferred by claustrophobic patients.
- Place arms at the sides or above the head, whichever is most comfortable for the patient. If you're using the gating option, place the arms by the sides to keep good blood flow to the fingers. Attach the P-gating device.
- Use accessories such as the knee bolster and blankets to make the patient as comfortable as possible.
- Locate T1 through T12 on the patient and determine which coils will best cover the whole spine (ex. CTL mid and CTL Bottom)
- Place the axial alignment light 2 cm above the xiphoid which is approximately T7. Press landmark
- Explicitly instruct the patient not to move during the scan, e.g: don't shift hips or move legs.

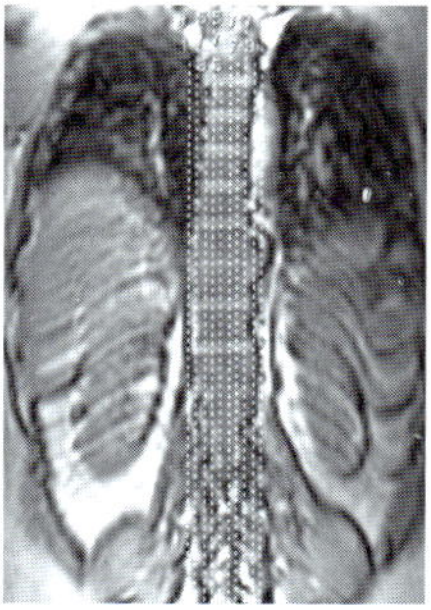

Coronal localizer for sagittal slices

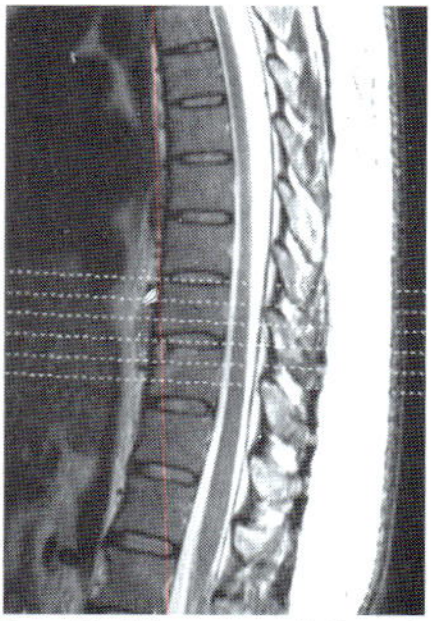

Sagittal image of the dorsal spine showing axial oblique slice positions parallel to each disk space

PROTOCOL: THORACIC SPINE

Indication

- Thoracic disc disease
- Thoracic cord compression
- Visualisation of an MS plaques in the thoracic cord
- Thoracic cord tumor
- To visualize the inferior extent of cervical syrinx

Sequences

Pulse Sequence	Sag - T2	Sag T1	Sag STIR	Axial-T2	Axial-T1	COR-T1
TR	3500	400'	3000	3000	350	500
TE/IR	102	Min	85/150	102	Min	13.0
ETL	16	—	8	32	2	2
Bandwidth	31.25	31.25	15.63	20.83	20.83	—
Nex	4	3	3	4	4	3
Slice	4	4	4	4	4	3
Gap	1	1	1	1	1	1
No. of Slices	11	11	10	11	11	9
Matrix Freq/Phase	384/256	512/224	256/192	256/256	256/224	384/256
FOV	36	36	36	22	22	36
SNR	100	100	100	100	100	100
Scan Time	3.51	4.35	3.42	3.24	2.34	3.14
Frequency Direction	A/P	A/P	S/I	A/P	Un swap	S/I
Auto Center Frequency	Water	Water	Water	Water	Water	Water
Flow Compensation Direction	Freq	—	—	Slice	—	—
Saturation	a,p	—	a,p	S,I		a

LUMBAR SPINE

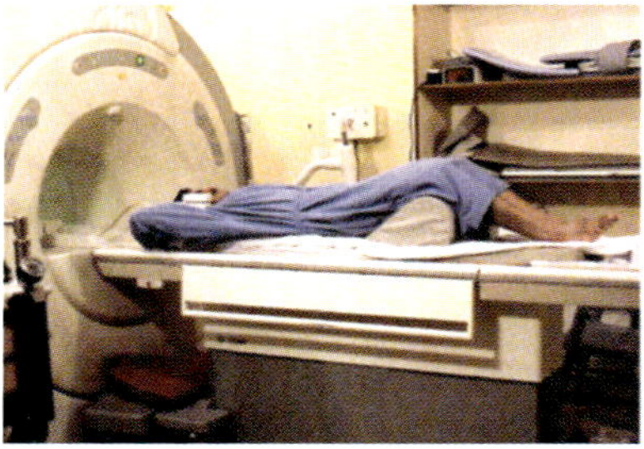

Patient Position-Phased Array Coil-CTL Bottom

- Place the phased array coil on the magnet table and plug the phased array coil port.
- Position patient supine and either head first.
- Place arms at the sides or above the head, whichever is most comfortable for the patient. If you're using the gating option, place the arms by the sides to keep good blood flow to the fingers. Attach the P-gating device. CTLBOT). Adjust the patient so that the anatomy of interest is center over the selected coil.
- Use accessories such as the knee bolster, to flatten the lumbar curve and bring it closer to the coil, and blankets to make the patient as comfortable as possible.

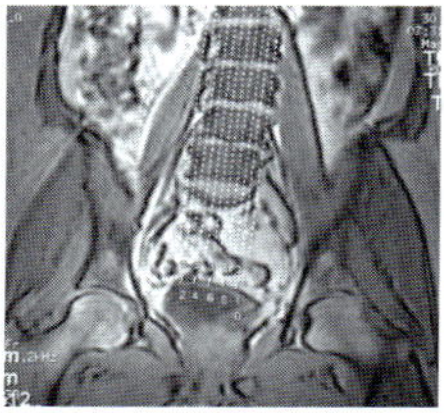

Coronal localizer for sagittal slices

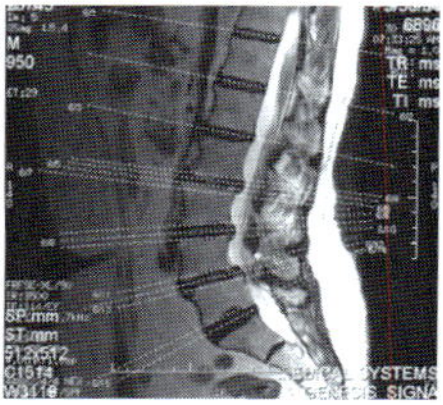

Sagittal image of the lumbar spine showing axial oblique slice prescription

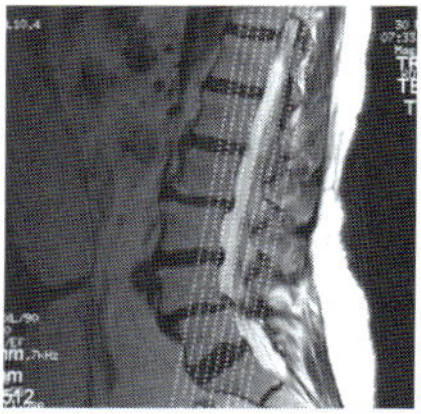

Sagittal localizer for coronal slices

PROTOCOL: LUMBAR SPINE

Indication

- Disc prolapse with cord or nerve root compression
- Spinal dysraphism to assess cord termination, syrinx, diastematomyelia
- Discitis
- Evaluation of the conus in patients with appropriate symptoms
- Arachnoiditis
- Arrange the form pads under the knees to elevate

Sequences

Pulse Sequence	Sag T2	Sag T1	Sag –STIR	Axial T2	Axial T1	Coronal T1
TR	3600	400	3000	3000	350	500
TE/IR	102	Min	50/150	102	Min	13
ETL	16	——	8	12	——	2
Bandwidth	20.83	31.25	15.63	20.83	31.25	——
Nex	4	3	3	3	3	3
Slice thickness	4	4	4	4	4	3
Gap	1	1	1	1	1	1
No. of Slices	11	11	11	11	11	9
Matrix Freq/Phase	256/224	512/224	256/224	256/224	512/192	384/256
FOV	28	28	28	20	20	36
SNR	100	87	100	93	88	100
Scan Time	3.29	3.28	4.18	2.57	3.22	3.14
Frequency Direction	A/P	A/P	A/P	A/P	A/P	A/P
Auto Center Frequency	Water	Water	Water	Water	Water	Water
Flow Compensation Direction	Slice	——	——	Slice	——	——
Saturation	L	L	——	S,I	S,I	a

WHOLE SPINE IMAGING

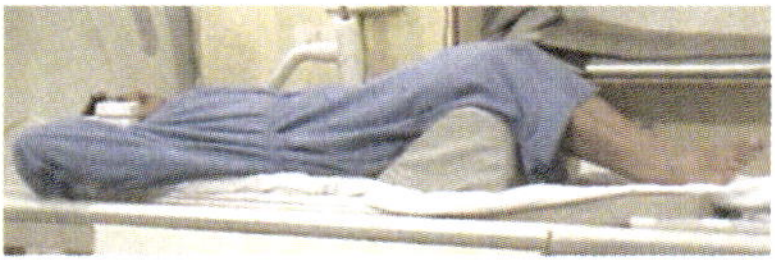

Patient Position-Phased Array Coil-CTL Mid

- Place the phased array coil on the magnet table and plug the phased array coil port.
- Position patient supine, and either head or feet first. A feet first position may be preferred by claustrophobic patients.
- Place arms at the sides or above the head, whichever is most comfortable for the patient. If you're using the gating option, place the arms by the sides to keep good blood flow to the fingers. Attach the P-gating device.
- Use accessories such as the knee bolster and blankets to make the patient as comfortable as possible.
- Locate C1-S1 on the patient and determine which coils will best cover the Whole spine (e.g. CTL mid and CTL Bottom)
- Explicitly instruct the patient not to move during the scan. e.g: don't shift hips or move legs.

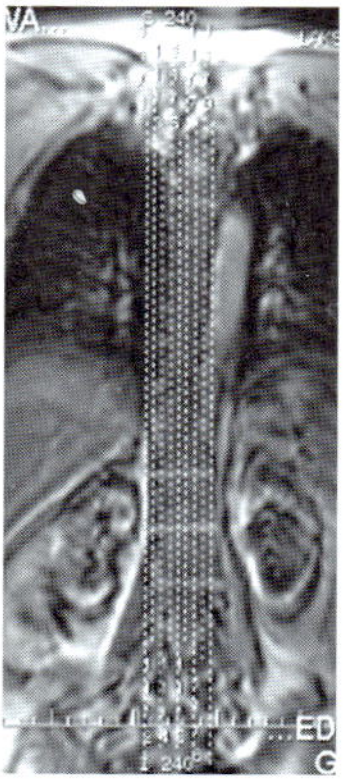

Coronal localizer for sagittal slices

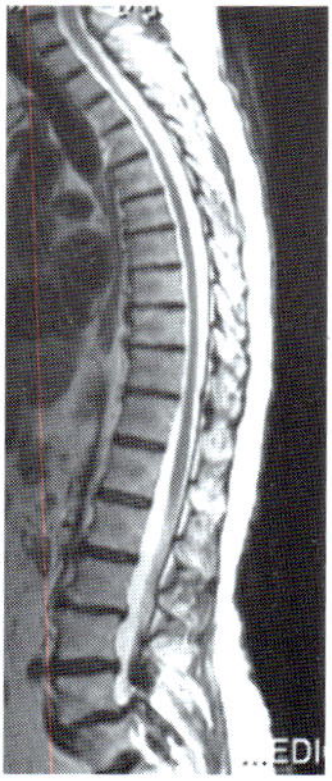

Sagittal spine showing axial oblique slice positions parallel to each disc spaces

PROTOCOL: WHOLE SPINE IMAGING

Indication

- Cord compression (level unknown) , due to metalistic disease or primary cord tumor
- Bone marrow screening
- Congenital abnormalities of spinal curvature (scoliosis and kyphosis)
- Evaluation of the extent of syrinx
- Heptomeningeal disease

Sequences

Pulse Sequence	Sag - T2	Sag T1	Sag STIR	Axial-T2	Axial-T1	COR-T1
TR	3500	400‘	3000	3000	350	500
TE/IR	102	Min	85/150	102	Min	13.0
ETL	16	——	8	32	2	2
Bandwidth	31.25	-31.25	15.63	20.83	20.83	——
Nex	4	3	3	4	4	3
Slice	4	4	4	4	4	3
Gap	1	1	1	1	1	1
No. of Slices	11	11	10	11	11	9
Matrix Freq/Phase	384/256	512/224	256/192	256/256	256/224	384/256
FOV	48	48	48	22	22	36
SNR	100	100	100	100	100	100
Scan Time	3.51	4.35	3.42	3.24	2.34	3.14
Frequency Direction	A/P	A/P	S/I	A/P	Un swap	S/I
Auto Center Frequency	Water	Water	Water	Water	Water	Water
Flow Compensation Direction	Freq	——	——	Slice	——	——
Saturation	a,p	——	a,p	S,I		a

CHEST

CHEST

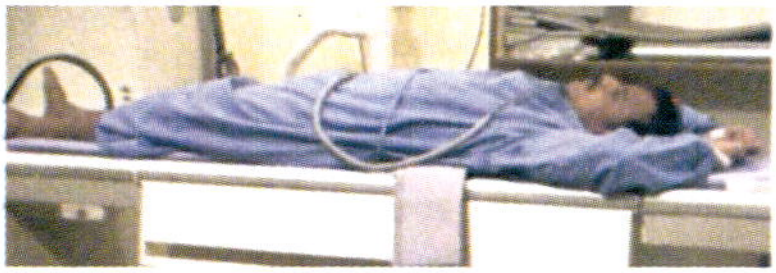

Placement of the gating leads

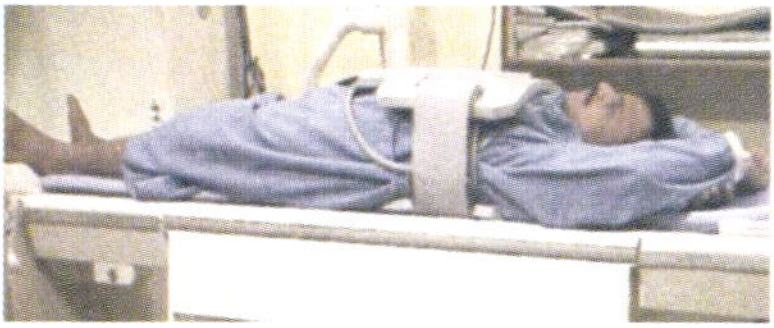

Patient position: Torso array coil
Place the patient supine, feet first on the table.

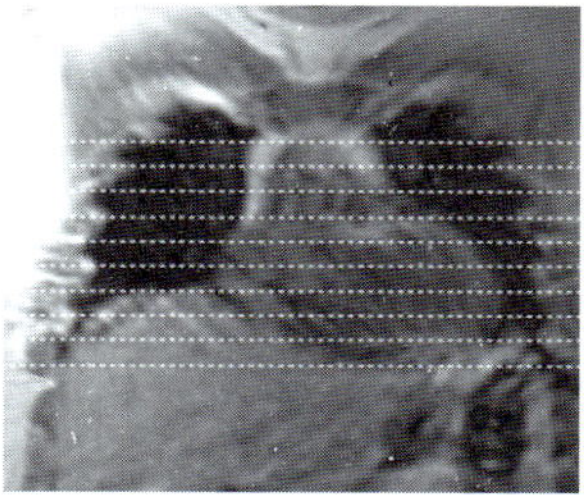

Coronal localizer for axial slices

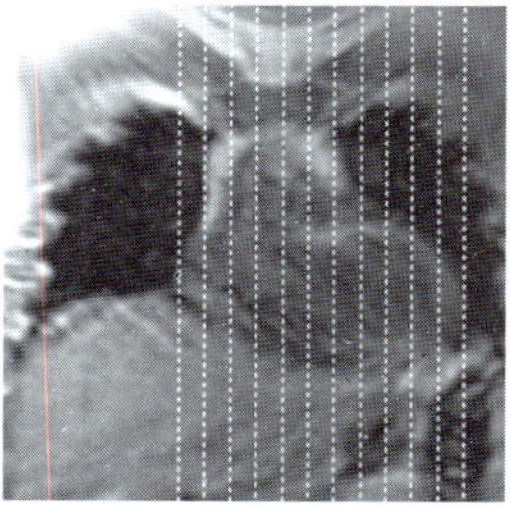

Coronal localizer for sagittal slices

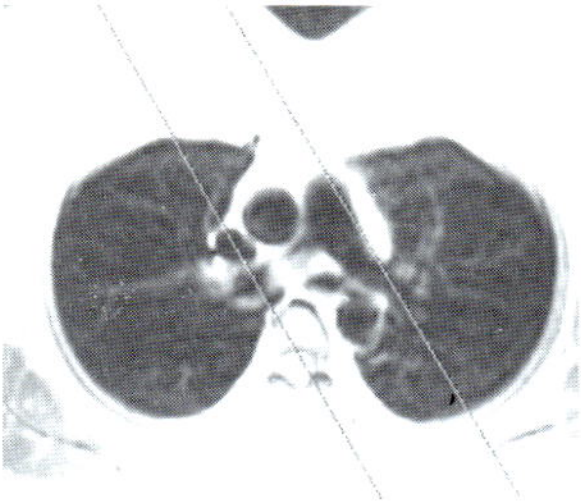

Axial image through the ascending and descending Aorta showing correct placement of the first and last oblique slices for examining the arch of aorta

PROTOCOL: CHEST

Indication

- Mediastinal mass, adenopathy

Sequences

Pulse Sequence	Axial SE	AXIAL FSE	Oblique Cine	Oblique Coronal T1 SE
TR	—	—	18	—
TE/IR	Minimum	14.0	Min	Minimum
ETL	—	12	FA30 Deg	—
Bandwidth	15.00	20.83	15.63	15.63
Nex	4.00	4.00	2.00	4.00
Slice	10	10	10	10
Gap	2	2	2	2
No. of Slices	20	20	20	16
Matrix Freq/Phase	256/128	256/128	256/128	256/128
FOV	32	32	32	32
SNR	100	100	100	100
Scan Time	8.54	4.54	2.36	8.54
Frequency Direction	R/L	R/L	Unswap	Unswap
Auto Center Frequency	Water	Water	Water	Water
Flow Compensation Direction	—	—	—	—
Saturation	S,I	S,I	—	—

Remarks:

- All sequences are cardiac gated.
- Set TR to 80% of R-R Interval for T1 weighted image, trigger every second or third R wave for T2 weighting

HEART AND GREAT VESSELS

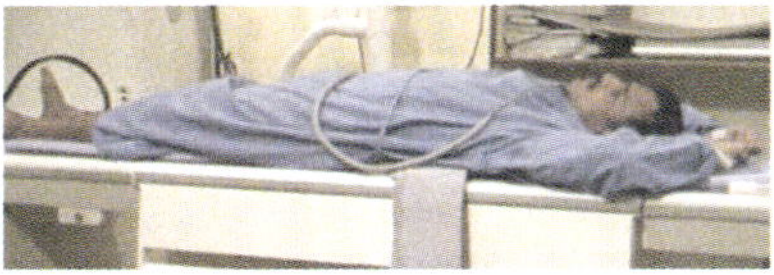

Placement of the gating leads bellows

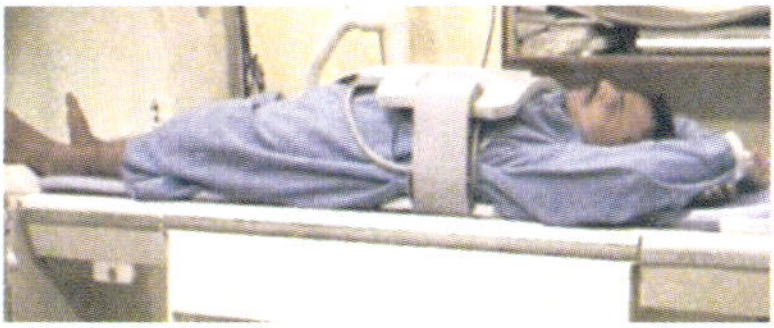

- Patient position-Torso array coil
- Place the patient supine, feet first on the table.

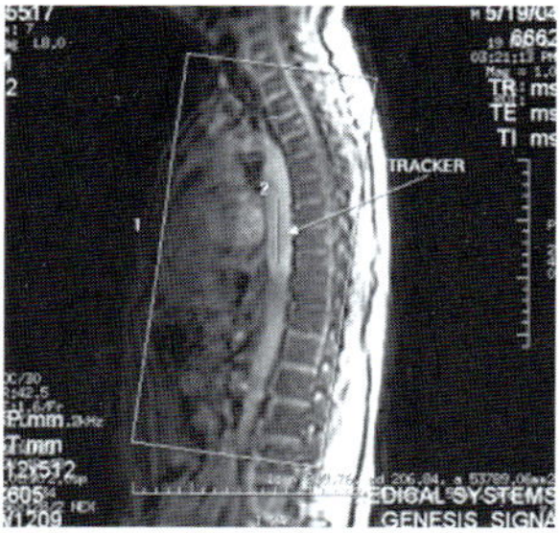

Sagittal localizer to obtain coronal images

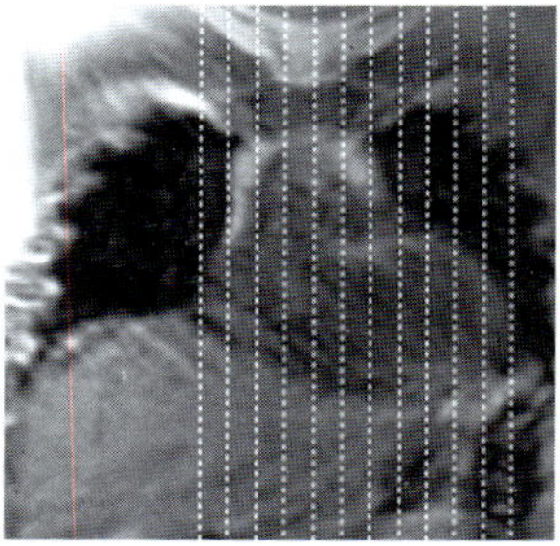

Coronal localizer for sagittal slices

PROTOCOL: HEART AND GREAT VESSELS

Indication

- Diagnosis and evaluation of thoracic aortic aneurysm, dissection and coarctation
- Assessment of complex congenital abnormalities of the heart and great vessels
- Diagnosis of atrial or ventricular septal defect
- Assessment of ventricular function
- Assessment of ventricular muscle mass
- Evaluation of vessel patency and thrombus
- Evaluation of valvular dysfunction

Sequences

Pulse Sequence	Vasc, TOF SPGR	Axial T1 FSE	Sagittal T2 FSE
TR	—	—	—
TE/IR	Minimum	Minimum	Minimum
ETL	FA-45deg	18	16
Bandwidth	31.25	20.83	20.83
Nex	1	3.00	3.00
Slice	2..8	4	4
Gap	30	5	5
No. of Slices	128	14	9
Matrix Freq/Phase	256/160	384/256	384/256
FOV	38	32	32
SNR	100	100	100
Scan Time	0.29	3.50	2.30
Frequency Direction	A/P	R/L	S/I
Auto Center Frequency	Water	Water	Water
Flow Compensation Direction	—	—	—
Saturation	—	—	—

Contrast Usage: 20 ml Bolus

Remarks:

- Select tracker button
- Save the series with tracker
- Smart prep
- Breath hold
- Placement of the gating leads (ECG)

BREAST

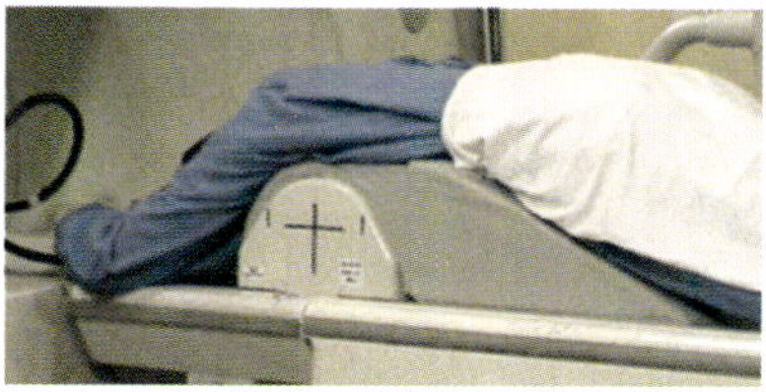

Patient Position: Breast coil

- Place the patient prone head first on the table.
- Place breast coil, cushions, and body pad with ankle pad on the table. Position the coil with the cable end pointing towards the magnet.
- Insert the appropriate pads into the coil wells.
- Lower the patient transport to its lowest position to help the patient position herself.
- Seat the patient on the table between the body pad and ankle support.

Patient Preparation Instructions

- Deodorant and nipple earrings may cause artifacts: have the patient remove both if necessary.
- Have the patient change into a gown with the opening in the front.
- Apply nipple markers if requested by the Radiologist Incorrect positioning compresses the nipple and distorts the overall breast shape

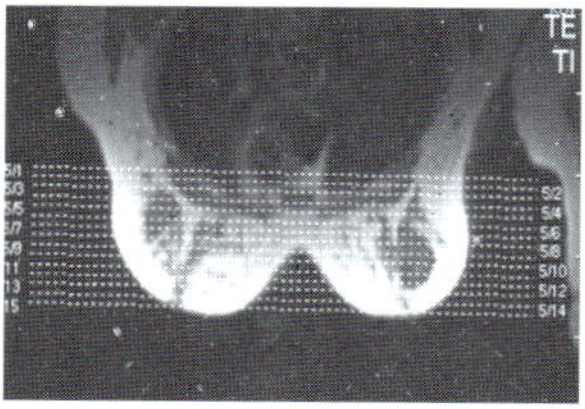

Axial localizer for coronal slices

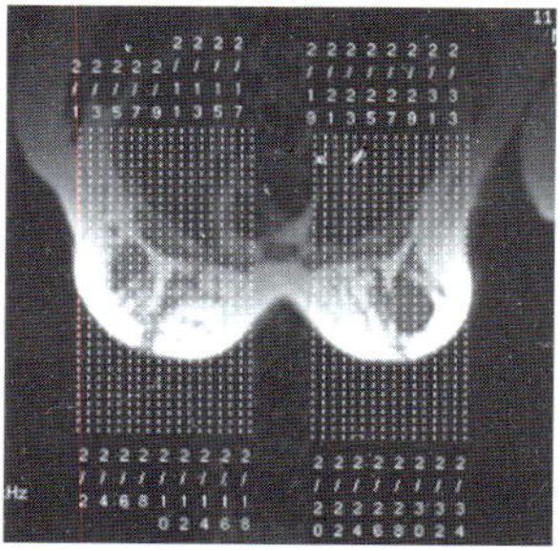

Axial localizer for sagittal slices

PROTOCOL: BREAST

Indication:

- Characterization of abnormalities seen on a mammogram especially , but not exclusively , in patients with previous disease
- Characterization of abnormalities in patients with very fatty breasts
- Characterization of abnormalities in patients with breast implants

Sequences

Pulse Sequence	Sag FSE T2	Sag FAST STIR Water SAT	Sag FAST STIR-FAT SAT	Axial-FSE T2	Axial T1 FSE	Axial T1 FAT SAT
TR	4200	4600	4600	4700	400	400
TE/IR	85.0	50/150	50/150	85.0	8.0	8.0
ETL	16	6	6	16	3	3
Bandwidth	20.83	15.63	15.63	20.83	31.25	31.25
Nex	4	2	2	4	4	4
Slice	5	5	5	5	4	4
Gap	1	1	1	1	1	1
No. of Slices	18	18	18	20	16	16
Matrix Freq/Phase	256/256	256/192	256/192	320/256	224/160	224/160
FOV	20	20	20	36	18	18
SNR	100	100	100	100	100	100
Scan Time	4.33	5.02	4.57	5.05	2.58	4.27
Frequency Direction	A/P	A/P	A/P	A/P	A/P	A/P
Auto Center Frequency	Water	Fat	Fat	Water	Water	Water
Flow Compensation Direction	—	—	—	—	—	—
Saturation	S,I	S,I, Water	S,I	S,I	S,I	S,I, FAT

BRACHIAL PLEXUS

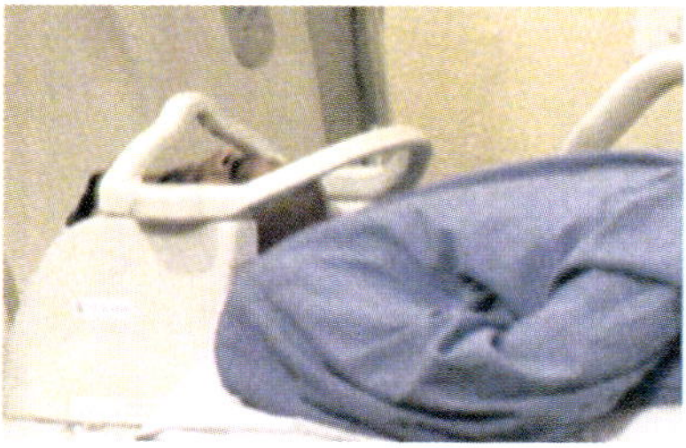

Patient Position-CTL top

- Place the coil on the magnet table and plug it in.
- Place patient supine, head first. Rest the head and neck in the coil.
- Position the superior end of the coil at the base of the skull. This position should include C1 on a sagittal image so that you can count vertebra for localization purpose.

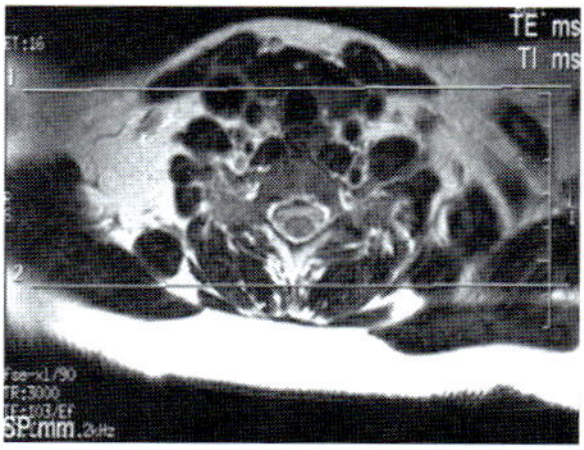

Axial localizer for Brachial Plexus showing correct Placement of the first and last slices of the coronal series

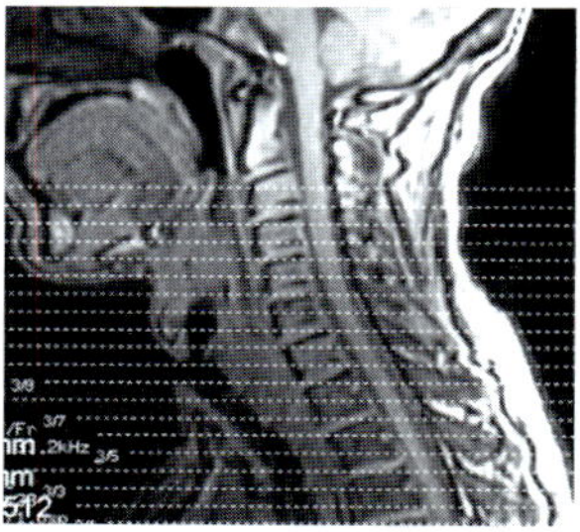

Sagittal localizer for axial slices

PROTOCOL: BRACHIAL PLEXUS

Indication

- Diagnosis and characterization of brachial plexus lesions, especially those secondary to carcinoma of the breast and the bronchus
- Thoracic outlet syndrome
- evaluation of the brachial plexus following trauma

Sequences

Pulse Sequence	Cor T2	Cor T1	Cor-STR	Sag T2-FSE	Sag-STIR	Axial T2
TR	3500	600	2700	3500	2700	3000
TE/IR	102	Min	50/150	102	50/150	102
ETL	16	2	6	16	6	16
Bandwidth	31.25	20.83	15.63	31.25	15.63	31.25
Nex	4	3	2	4	2	4
Slice	4	4	4	3	3	4
Gap	1	1	1	1	1	3
No. of Slices	14	11	10	15	11	12
Matrix Freq/Phase	384/256	384/256	384/256	384/256	256/192	256/192
FOV	32	32	32	34	24	22
SNR	100	100	106	100	100	100
Scan Time	3.51	3.53	3.57	3.51	2.58	2.30
Frequency Direction	Unswap	Unswap	R/L	Swap	R/L	S/I
Auto Center Frequency	Water	Water	Water	Water	Water	Water
Flow Compensation Direction	Freq	—	—	—	—	Slice
Saturation	A,p	A,P	—	A,P	—	—

ABDOMINAL ANGIO

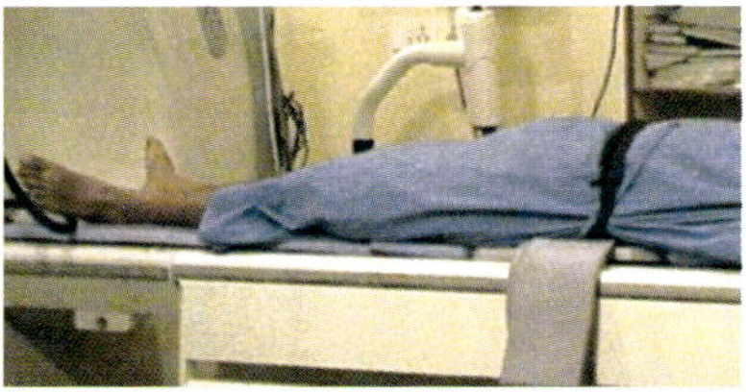

Placement of the respiratory compensation (RC) bellows

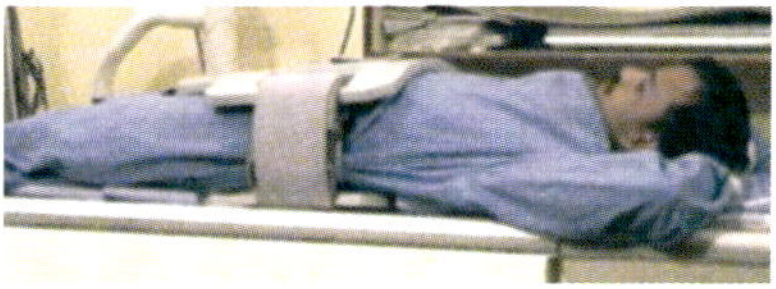

Patient Position- Torso array coil

- Position the patient supine, feet first
- Place the arms at the sides or overhead.
- Position comfort cushions at any pressure points, e.g. under elbows.

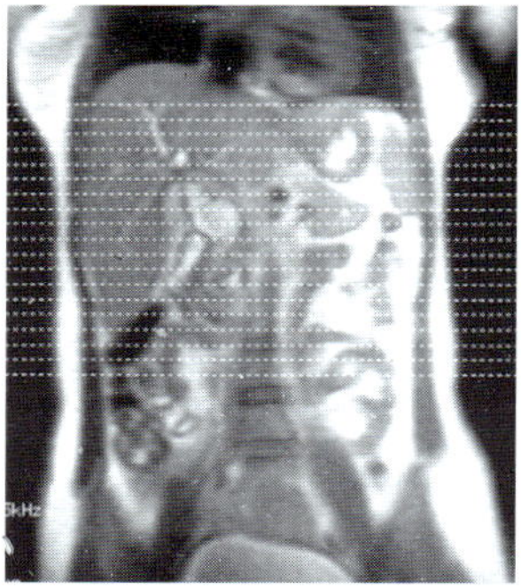

Coronal localizer for axial slices

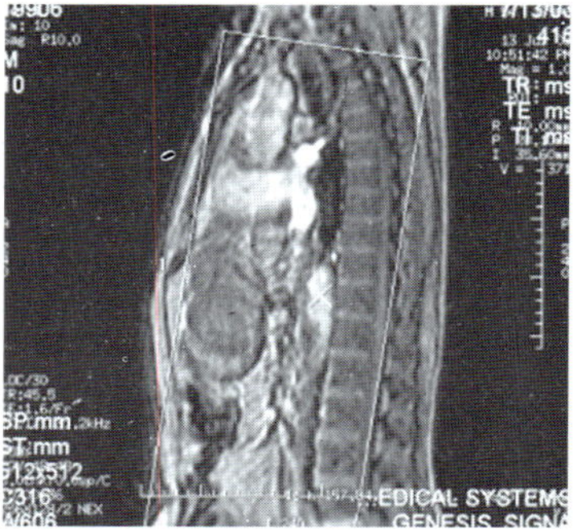

Sagittal localizer to obtain coronal slices

PROTOCOL: ABDOMEN- VASCULAR IMAGING

Indication

- Preoperative assessment of abdominal aortic aneurysyms
- Demonstration of major vascular anatomy
- Evaluation of hepatic vascular anatomy prior to tumor resection
- Assessment of renal vein thrombosis
- Assessment of vasculature prior to renal transplant

Sequences

Pulse Sequence	Vasc. ToF, SpGR	Axial T1 FSE	Sagittal T1 FSE
TR	—	—	—
TE/IR	Minimum	Minimum	Minimum
ETL	FA-45Deg	18	16
Bandwidth	31.25	20.83	20.83
Nex	1	3	3
Slice	2.6	4	4
Gap	36	5	5
No. of Slices	128	14	9
Matrix Freq/Phase	256/160	384/256	384/256
FOV/Phase FOV	48/.80	32	32
SNR	100	100	100
Scan Time	0.29	3.50	2.30
Frequency Direction	A/P	R/L	S/I
Auto Center Frequency	Water	Water	Water
Flow Compensation Direction	—	—	—
Saturation	—	—	—

Contrast Usage: 20 ml Bolus

Remarks:

- Select tracker button
- Save the series with tracker
- Smart prep
- Breath hold

MRCP

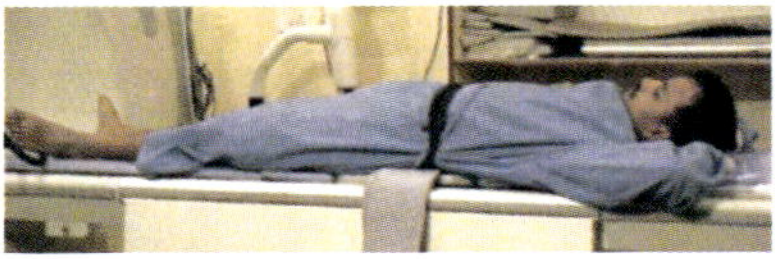

Placement of the respiratory compensation (RC) bellows

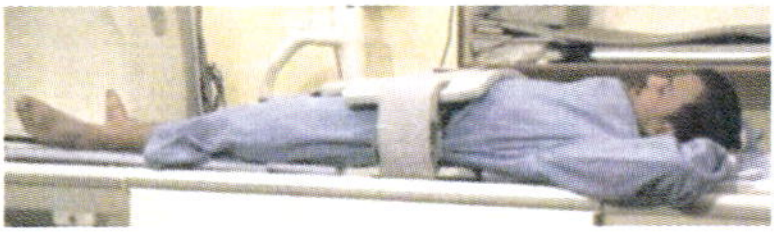

Patient Position: Torso phased array coil

- Position the patient supine, feet first on the table.
- Place the arms at the sides or under the head.

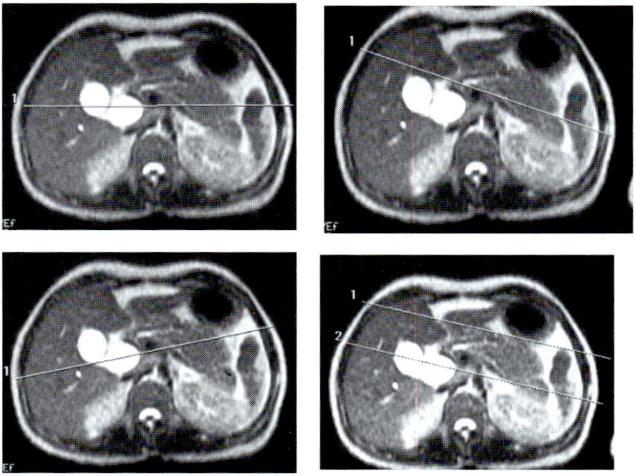

SSFSE- single shot breath hold technique

PROTOCOL: MRCP

Indication

- For the evaluation of biliary system in cases of obstructive jaundice
- Pancreas divisum
- For the evaluation of intrahepatic biliary ducts in the postoperative conditions
- For the evaluation of pancreatic duct abnormalities

Sequences

Pulse Sequence	Axial SPGR T1	Axial SSFSE T2	Thick Slab	Thin Slab	Thinner Slices
TR	140	1069	2045	2045	2045
TE/IR	Minimum	90	Maximum	Maximum	Maximum
ETL	90	—	—	—	—
Bandwidth	31.25	62.50	31.25	31.25	31.25
Nex	1	—	—	—	—
Slice	10	8	70	40	4.0
Gap	2.0	2	0	0	0
No. of Slices	16	20	1	1	12
Matrix Freq/Phase	256/192	256/128	512/256	384/256	384/256
FOV	40	40	36	40	40
SNR	100	100	100	100	100
Scan Time	0.21	0.20	0.01	0.01	0.23
Frequency Direction	R/L	R/L	Unswap	A/P	S/I
Auto Center Frequency	Water	Water	Water	Water	Water
Flow Compensation Direction	—	—	—	—	—
Saturation	—	—	—	—	—

MRU

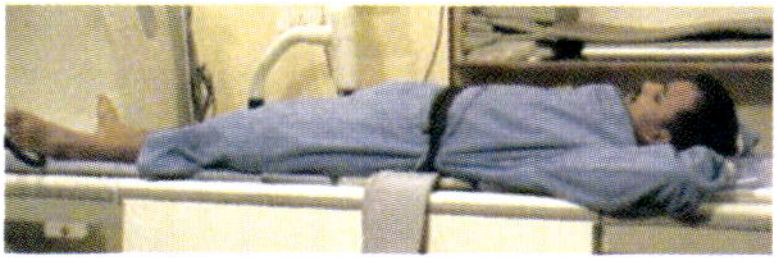

Placement of the RC bellows

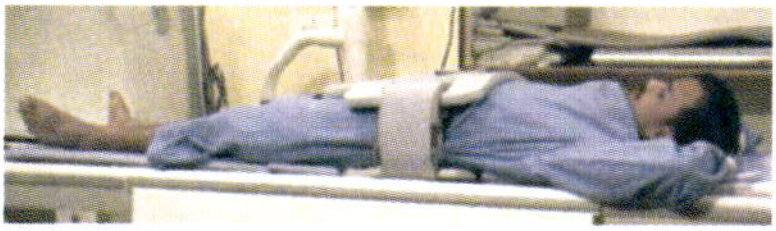

Patient Position: Torso array coil

- Position the patient supine, feet first on the table.
- Place the arms at the sides or under the head.

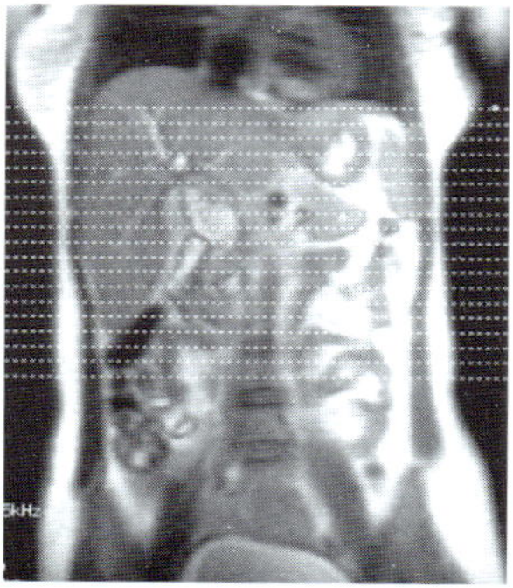

Coronal localizer for axial slices

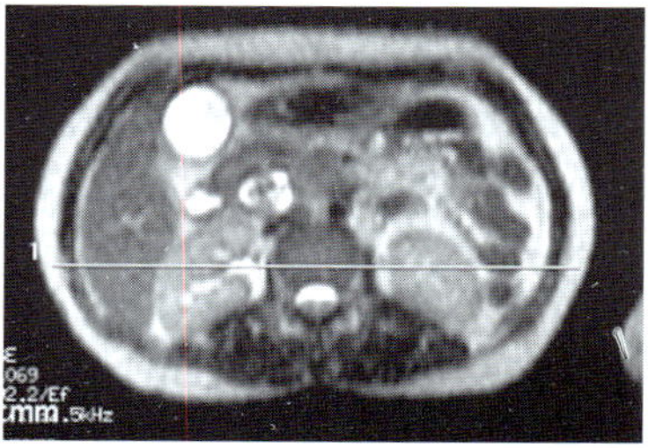

Axial localizer to obtain MRU slab

PROTOCOL: MRU

Indication

- For the evaluation of urinary tract in patients with renal failure
- For the evaluation of non-excreting kidneys in IVU
- For the evaluation of urinary obstruction

Sequences

Pulse Sequence	MRU Thick Slab	MRU Thin Slab	MRU Thinner Slab	Axial SSFSE T2
TR	2045	2045	2045	1069
TE/IR	883	883	883	90
ETL	—	—	—	—
Bandwidth	31.25	31.25	31.25	62.50
Nex	—	—	—	—
Slice	70	40	4	8
Gap	0	0	0	2
No. of Slices	1	1	20	20
Matrix Freq/Phase	256/256	256/256	256/256	256/128
FOV	40	40	40	40
SNR	100	100	100	100
Scan Time	0.01	0.01	0.39	0.20
Frequency Direction	S/I	Unswap	S/I	R/L
Auto Center Frequency	Water	Water	Water	Water
Flow Compensation Direction	—	—	—	—
Saturation	—	—	—	—

PELVIS

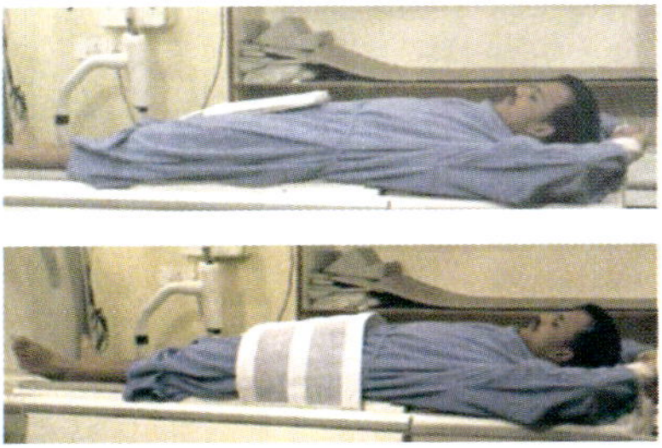

Patient Position- Pelvic Array Coil

Patient Preparation:

- An empty bladder can minimize motion artifacts from urine. However, a full bladder can aid visualization of bladder wall anatomy and pathology by improving definition between anatomy, (e.g. differentiating prostate from bladder wall).

Patient Position:

- Position the patient supine, feet first. Place an angle sponge under the knee for comfort.
- Place the arms at the or overhead.
- Position comfort cushions at any pressure points (e.g. under elbow)

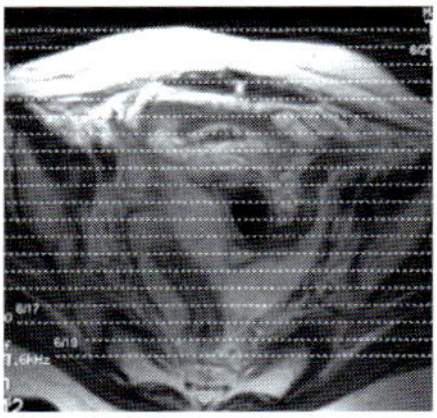

Axial localizer for coronal slices

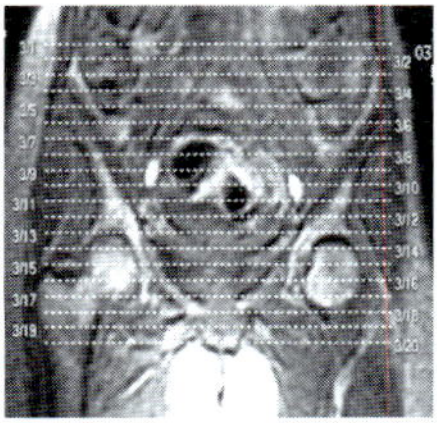

Coronal localizer for axial slices

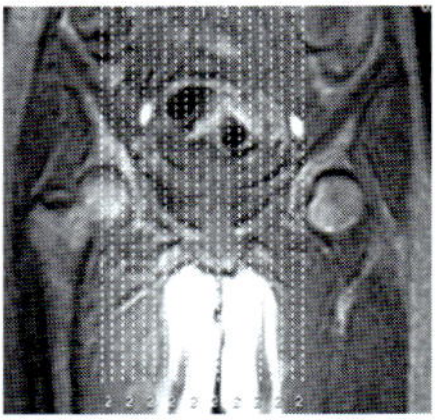

Coronal localizer for sagittal slices

PROTOCOL: PELVIS

Indication

- Assessment of congenital abnormalities of the urogenital tract
- Diagnosis and staging of carcinoma of the cervix
- Diagnosis of carcinoma of the uterus
- Assessment of benign uterine tumours, e.g: Leiomyoma and fibroids
- Diagnosis of carcinoma of the bladder rectum
- Evaluation of rectal fistulae especially in patients with Crohn's disease
- Evaluation of sacral lesions.

Sequences

Pulse Sequence	Sag FSE T2	Axial FSE T2	Axial SE T1	Cor FSE T2	Cor FSE IR	Cor FSE T2 fat sat
TR	5000	4500	675	4650	4775	5000
TE/IR	102.0	80	Min	80	50/150	102
ETL	12	21	—	21	6	10
Bandwidth	15.63	31.25	20.83	31.25	20.83	15.63
Nex	3	3	2	3	2	3
Slice	5	8	8	5	5	4
Gap	1	2	2	1	1	1
No. of Slices	20	20	20	20	20	20
Matrix Freq/Phase	320/256	256/256	256/192	256/256	256/192	320/256
FOV	24	38	38	38	38	24
SNR	100	100	100	100	100	100
Scan Time	5.35	3.13	4.17	3.05	5.09	5.35
Frequency Direction	A/P	R/L	R/L	S/I	S/I	S/I
Auto Center Frequency	Water	Water	Water	Water	Water	Water
Flow Compensation Direction	—	—	—	—	Freq	—
Saturation	S,I	S,I	S,I	S,I	S,I	S,I , FAT

ENDORECTAL

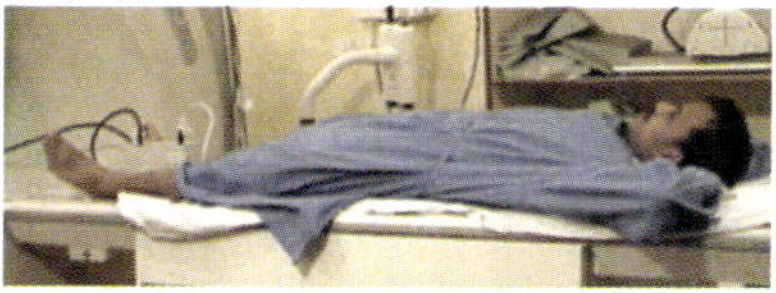

Patient Position- Endorectal coil

- Position the patient supine, feet first on the table.
- Place the arms at the side or under the head.
- Position comfort cushions at any pressure point, e.g. under elbows.

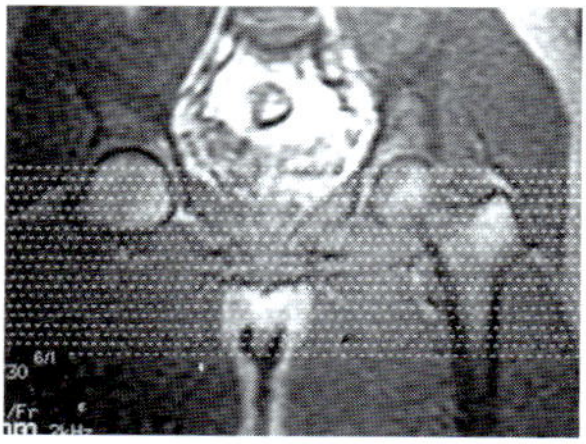

Coronal localizer for axial slices

PROTOCOL: ENDORECTAL

Indication

- Prostatic inflammation, benign hyperplasia and neoplasm

Sequences

Pulse Sequence	Sag FSE T2	Axial FSE T2	Axial SE T1	Axial STIR	Axial FSPGR T1 fat sat
TR	3525	3500	500	3000	175
TE/IR	102	102	Minimum	68/150	In phase
ETL	12	12	—	8	FA-60deg
Bandwidth	62.50	62.50	15.63	15.63	15.63
Nex	4	3	2	2	2
Slice	4	4	4	4	3
Gap	1	1	1	1	0.5
No. of Slices	20	20	19	10	30
Matrix Freq/Phase	256/256	256/256	256/192	256/192	256/192
FOV	16	16	16	16	16
SNR	100	100	100	100	100
Scan Time	5.17	3.58	3.20	2.30	4.39
Frequency Direction	S/I	R/L	R/L	A/P	R/L
Auto Center Frequency	Water	Water	Water	Water	Water
Flow Compensation Direction	—	Slice	—	—	—
Saturation	—	S,I	S,I	—	S,I fat

UPPER EXTREMITY

SHOULDER

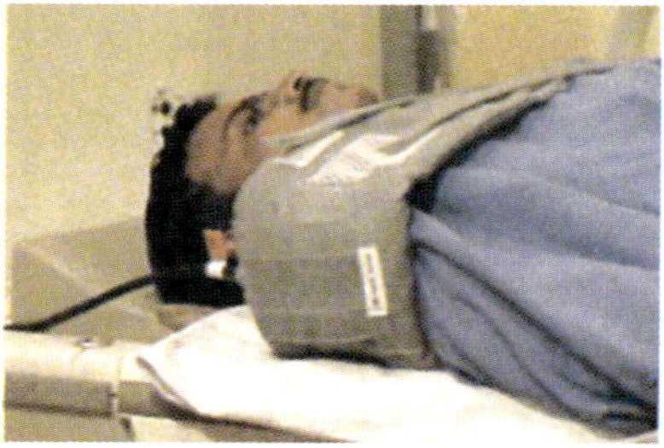

Patient Position-Flex coil

- Position the patient supine, head first. Offset the patient left or right and bring the shoulder as close as possible to magnet isocenter. To help minimize motion, oblique the patient, shoulder of interest down.
- Recheck the straps to make sure they are secure, now that the patient is lying down. Position the straps as far superior as possible to minimize respiratory motion.

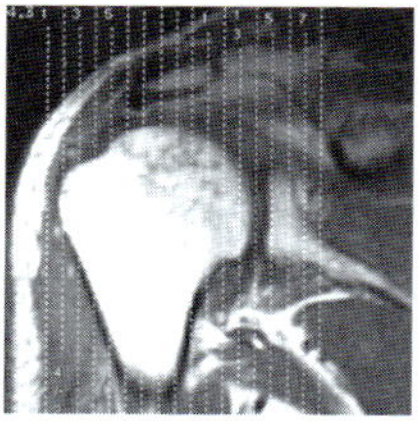

Coronal localizer for sagittal slices

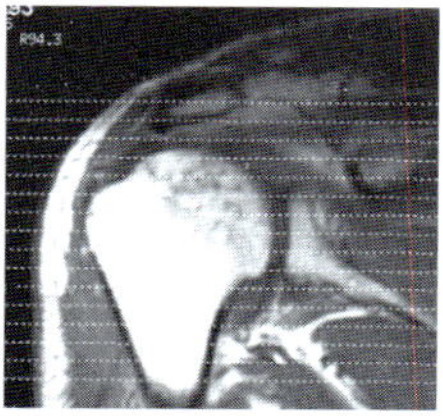

Coronal localizer for axial slices

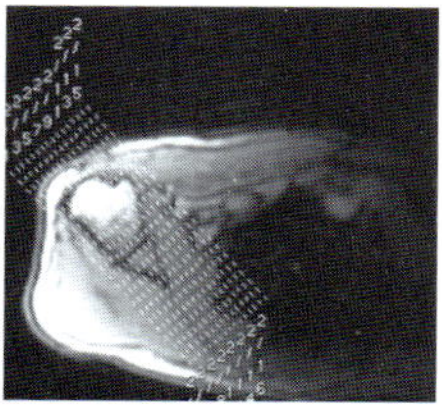

Axial localizer to obtain oblique coronal slices

PROTOCOL: SHOULDER

Indication

- Diagnosis and evaluation of impingement syndrome and instability
- Sometimes useful in the evaluation of frozen shoulder syndrome

Sequences

Pulse Sequence	Cor T1	Cor T2	Cor STIR-FSE	Sag T1 FSE	AX T1	AX T2* GRE
TR	500	3600	2600	500	500	500
TE/IR	Min	85.0	42/150	Min	Min	22.0
ETL	—	18	4	—	—	FA-20Dge.
Bandwidth	15.63	20.83	15.63	15.63	12.50	10.42
Nex	3	4	2	2	3	3
Slice	4	4	4	4	4	4
Gap	0	0	0	0	0	0
No. of Slices	16	14	12	12	12	12
Matrix Freq/Phase	256/256	256/256	256/192	256/224	256/256	256/224
FOV	14	14	14	14	14	12
SNR	100	100	100	100	100	100
Scan Time	6.32	3.43	4.15	3.52	6.32	5.40
Frequency Direction	Unswap	Uswap	Unswap	Unswap	R/L	R/L
Auto Center Frequency	Water	Water	Water	Water	Water	Water
Flow Compensation Direction	—	—	—	—	—	—
Saturation	R,I	R,I		R,I	R,I	R

Remarks: Both shoulders should be scanned for evaluation of symmetry.

HUMERUS

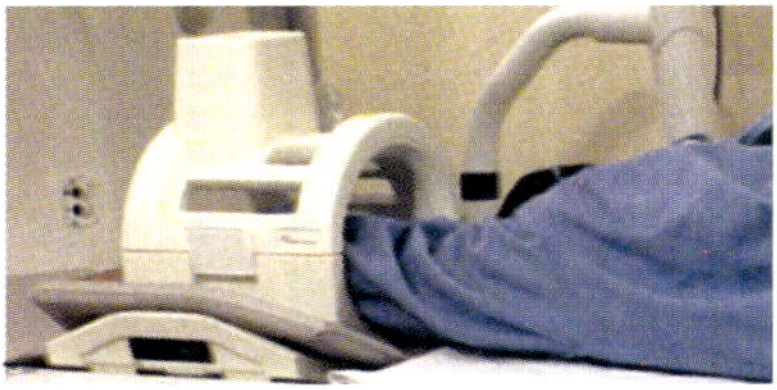

Patient Position: Extremity coil (Swimmer position)

- Position the patient prone, head first, arms at the sides
- Wrap the coil around the affected forearm with the cable end towards the magnet
- Turn on the alignment lights and landmark to centre of coil

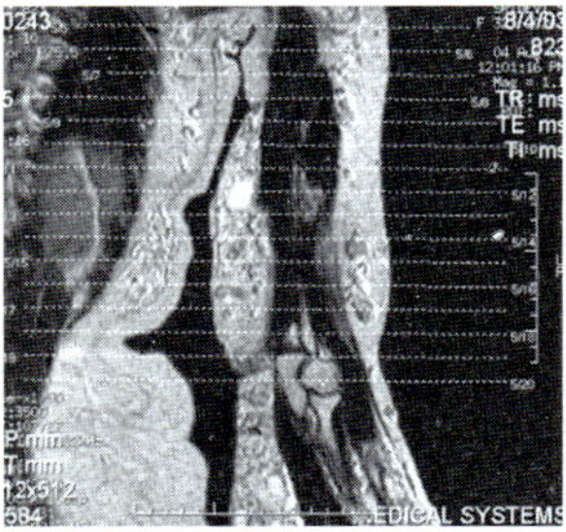

Coronal localizer for axial slices

PROTOCOL: HUMERUS

Indication

- Visualisation of bony and soft tissue abnormalities

Sequences

Pulse Sequence	O-CorT2 FSE	O-Axial T1 SE	Cor T2* GRE	O-Cor T1 SE	O-Axial STIR	O-Axial T2 FSE
TR	4000	550	550	450	2700	5075
TE/IR	85	Minimum	15	Minimum	85/150	85
ETL	16	—	FA-20Deg	—	6	16
Bandwidth	20.83	15.63	31.25	20.83	15.63	20.83
Nex	2	2	3	3.00	2	3
Slice	4	4	4	4	4	4
Gap	0	1	1	1	1	1
No. of Slices	16	16	16	16	10	16
Matrix Freq/Phase	384/160	256/224	512/256	512/256	256/192	384/256
FOV	16	16	16	16	12	16
SNR	100	100	100	100	100	100
Scan Time	1.28	4.09	6.28	5.45	2.58	4.08
Frequency Direction	A/P	S/I	Unswap	Unswap	Unswap	Unswap
Auto Center Frequency	Water	Water	Water	Water	Water	Water
Flow Compensation Direction	—	—	—	—	—	—
Saturation	a,p	—	—	—	—	—

ELBOW

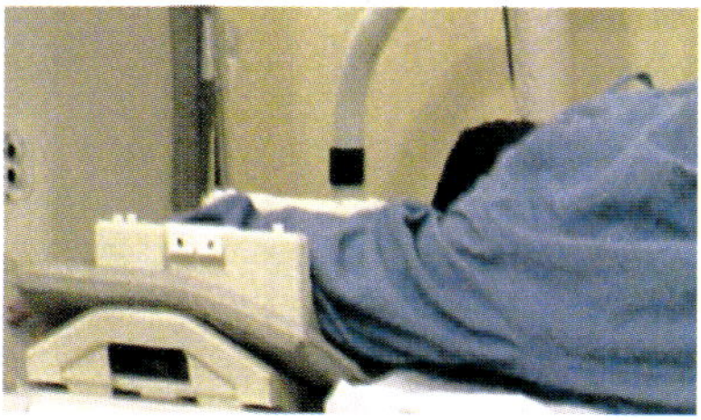

Patient Position: Extremity coil (Swimmer position)

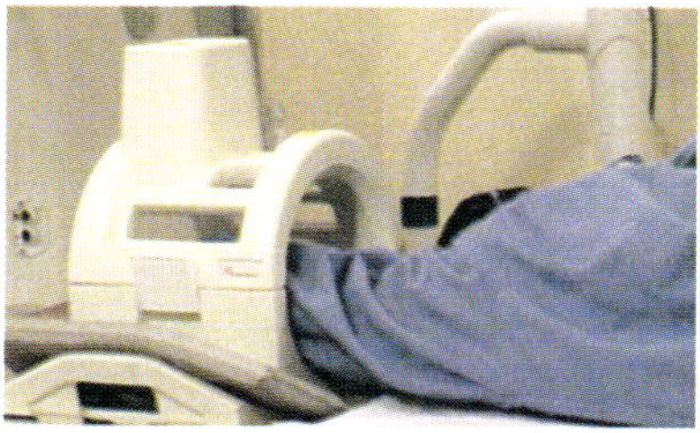

Patient Position: Extremity coil (Swimmer position)

- Position the patient prone, head first, arms at the sides.
- Wrap the coil around the affected forearm with the cable end towards the magnet.
- Do not overlap the coil, if the elbow is small, place the cushions around the forearm to keep the elbow centered in the flex coil.
- Turn on the alignment lights and landmark to centre of coil.

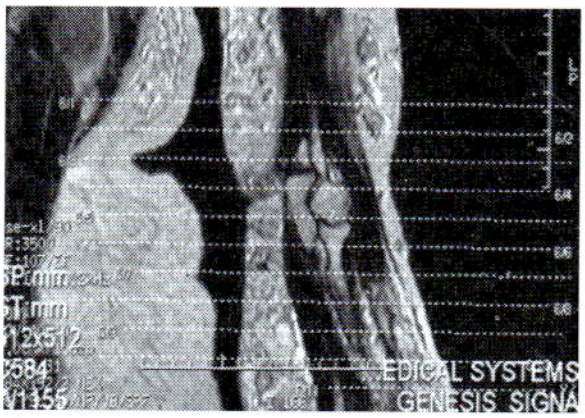

Coronal localizer for axial slices

PROTOCOL: ELBOW

Indication

- Visualisation of joint abnormalities
- Adjoining soft tissues(including bursa)

Sequences

Pulse Sequence	Cor T2	Cor STIR	CorT2* GRE	Sag T1	Sag STIR	Sag T2
TR	5075	2700	500	550	2700	5075
TE/IR	85	85.0/150	15	Min	85.0/150	85
ETL	85/16	6	FA-20Deg	—	6	16
Bandwidth	20.83	15.63	31.25	15.63	15.63	20.83
Nex	3	2	3	2	2	3
Slice	4	4	4	4	4	4
Gap	1	1	1	1	1	1
No. of Slices	20	20	20	20	10	10
Matrix Freq/Phase	384/256	256/192	512/256	256/224	256/192	384/256
FOV	16	12	16	16	12	16
SNR	100	100	100	100	100	100
Scan Time	4.08	2.58	628	4.09	2.58	4.08
Frequency Direction	A/P	S/I	Unswap	S/I	S/I	S/I
Auto Center Frequency	Water	Water	Water	Water	Water	Water
Flow Compensation Direction	—	—	—	—	—	—
Saturation	—	—	—	—	—	—

FOREARM

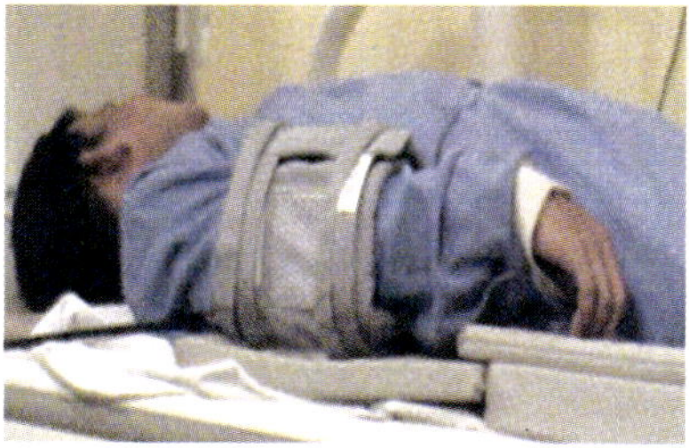

Patient Position-Flex coils

- Position the patient supine, head first, arms at the sides.
- Wrap the coil around the affected forearm with the cable end towards the magnet.
- Do not overlap the coil, if the forearm is small, place the cushions around the forearm to keep the forearm centered in the flex coil
- Turn on the alignment lights and landmark to centre of coil

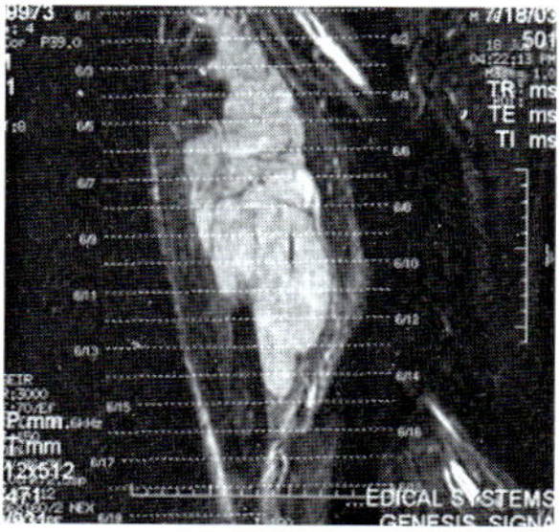

Coronal localizer for axial slices

PROTOCOL: FOREARM

Indication

- Visualization of bony and soft tissue abnormalities

Sequences

Pulse Sequence	O-CorT2 FSE	Cor T1 SE	O-Axial GRE	O-Axial SE	O-Cor T2 STIR	O-Axial T2 FSE
TR	4000	550	550	450	2700	5075
TE/IR	85	Minimum	15	Minimum	85/150	85
ETL	16	—	FA-20Deg	—	6	16
Bandwidth	20.83	15.63	31.25	20.83	15.63	20.83
Nex	2	2	3	3.00	2	3
Slice	4	4	4	4	4	4
Gap	0	1	1	1	1	1
No. of Slices	16	16	16	16	10	16
Matrix Freq/Phase	384/160	256/224	512/256	512/256	256/192	384/256
FOV	16	16	16	16	12	16
SNR	100	100	100	100	100	100
Scan Time	1.28	4.09	6.28	5.45	2.58	4.08
Frequency Direction	A/P	S/I	Unswap	Unswap	Unswap	Unswap
Auto Center Frequency	Water	Water	Water	Water	Water	Water
Flow Compensation Direction	—	—	—	—	—	—
Saturation	a,p	—	—	—	—	—

WRIST AND HAND

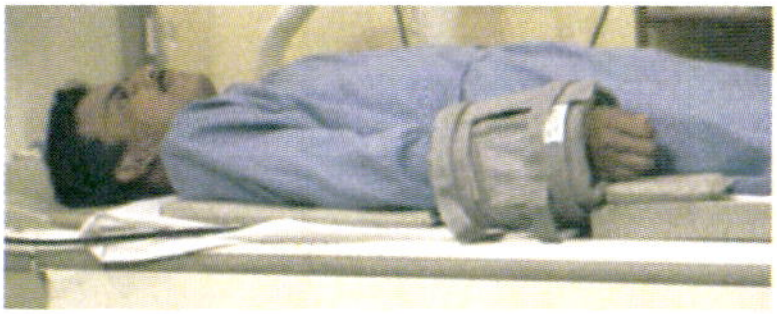

Patient Position: Flex coil

- Place the coil on the table and plug it into the surface coil port
- Position the patient supine, arm at the side with the wrist either prone (palm down) or lateral (thumb up).

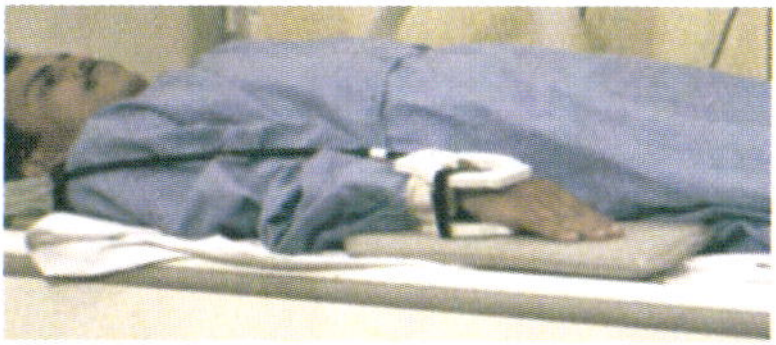

Patient Position: 3" coils in a dual

- Place the wrist prone, with the carpal bones positioned in the coil center of one coil. Place the other coil on top of the wrist and secure it with straps.
- Do not place the two coils facing one another, rather, position them back-to-back.

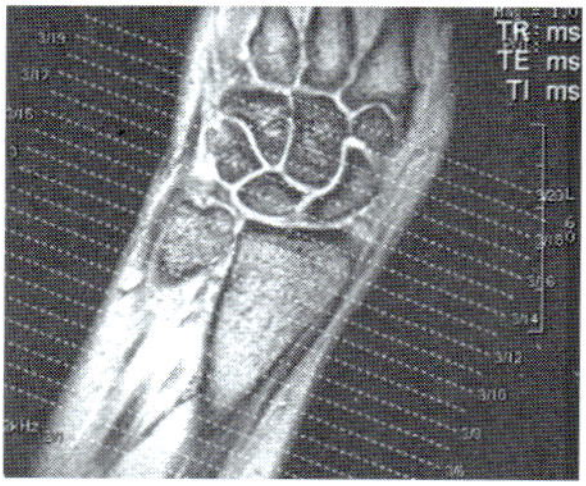

Coronal localizer for axial slices

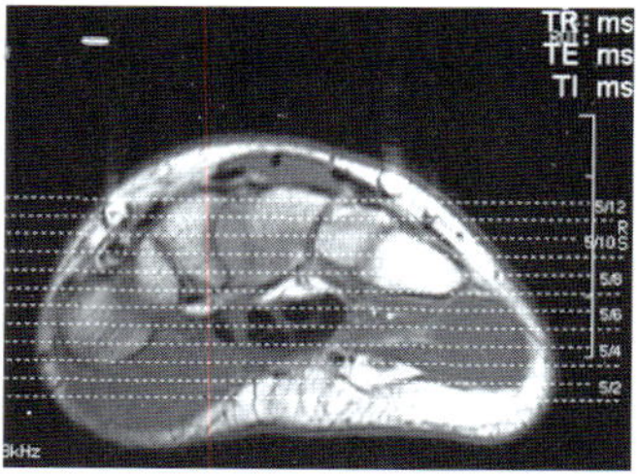

Axial localizer for coronal slices

PROTOCOL: WRIST AND HAND

Indication

- Assessment of wrist pain of unknown origin, (tears of the triangular cartilage) osteronecrosis of the lunate, occult ganglia
- Assessment of avascular necrosis (AVN) of the scaphoid following trauma
- Diagnosis of carpal tunnel syndrome/ tenosynovitis
- Possibly valuable in early evaluation of rheumatoid arthritis
- Assessment of the scapholunate and scaphotriquetral ligament when wrist instability is suspected.

Sequences

Pulse Sequence	COR T1SE	O-COR T2 FSE	O-COR T2*GRE	Oblique STIR	O-Axial T1 SE	Oblique PD
TR	550	5075.0	500	3000	450	3000
TE/IR	Minimum	85.0	15.0	150/50	Minimum	30.0
ETL	—	16	Flip Ang-20 deg	8	—	7
Bandwidth	15.63	20.83	31.25	15.63	20.83	25
Nex	2	3	3	2	3	3
Slice	4	4	4	3	4	2
Gap	1.0	1	1	0	1	0.2
No. of Slices	16	20	20	11	20	20
Matrix Freq/Phase	256/224	384/256	512/256	256/192	512/256	256/192
FOV	16	16	16	12	16	10
SNR	100	100	100	100	100	100
Scan Time	4.09	4.08	6.28	2.30	5.45	4.18
Frequency Direction	A/P	A/P	Unswap	Unswap	Unswap	A/P
Auto Center						
Frequency	Water	Water	Water	Water	Water	Water
Flow Compensation Direction	—	—	—	—	—	—
Saturation	I	—	—	S,I	—	—

Remarks: Both wrists should be scanned for evaluation of symmetry.

LOWER EXTREMITY

HIPS

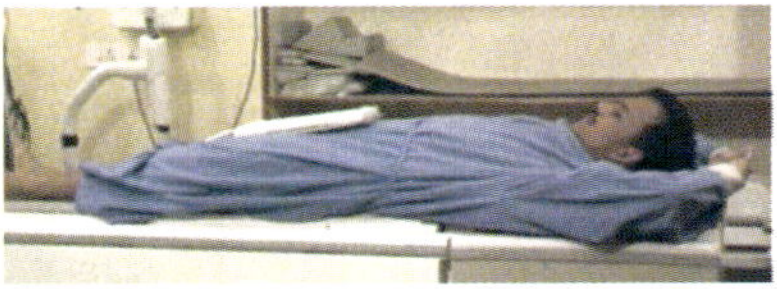

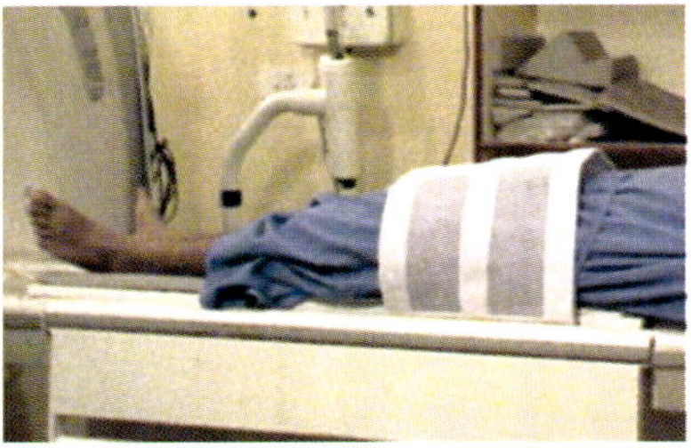

Patient Position-Pelvic array coil

- Place the pelvic array coil on the table.
- Place the patient supine, feet first, with the legs extended and straight.
- Place the patient's arms at the sides or resting on the abdomen, but not on the pelvis.
- Position comfort cushions at any pressure points.
- If necessary, use patient straps to immobilize the patient and provide support for the arms. Tape the feet together so the legs and hips are immobilized.

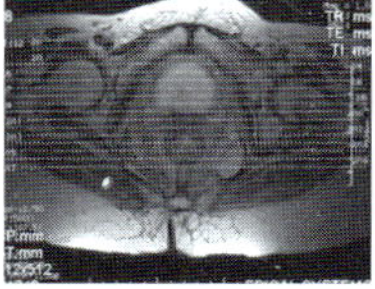

Axial localizer for coronal slices

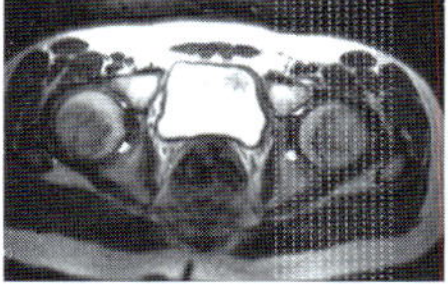

Axial localizer for sagittal slices

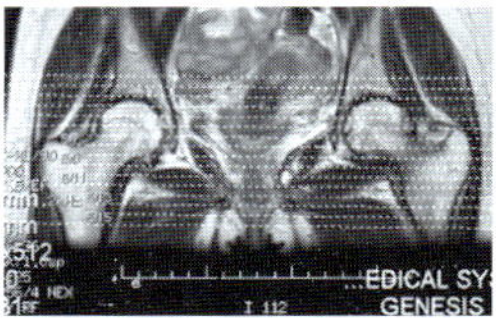

Coronal localizer for axial slices

PROTOCOL: HIPS

Indication

- Evaluation of unexplained hip pain mainly caused by avascular necrosis(AVN) of the femoral head
- Possibly useful in the diagnosis of labral tears

Sequences

Pulse Sequence	O/Cor FSE T2	O/Cor SE T1	O/Cor FAST STIR	O/Cor GRE T2*	O/AX-SET1	Axail FSE T2
TR	4825.0	525	3000	500	525	5000
TE/IR	85	Min. Full	50/150	20.0	Min. Full	102.0
ETL	16	—	6	FA-20 deg	—	12
Bandwidth	20.83	31.25	15.63	15.63	31.25	15.63
Nex	4	3	2	3	3	3
Slice	4	4	4	4	4	5
Gap	1	1	1	1	1	1
No. of Slices	16	16	12	16	16	20
Matrix Freq/Phase	448/224	512/192	256/192	256/192	512/192	320/256
FOV	32	32	32	32	36	24
SNR	100	100	100	100	100	100
Scan Time	4.34	5.06	3.18	4.52	3.51	5.35
Frequency Direction	Unswap	Unswap	Unswap	A/P	Unswap	A/P
Auto Center Frequency	Water	Water	Water	Water	Water	Water
Flow Compensation Direction	—	—	—	—	—	—
Saturation	I	S,I	—	S,I	S,I	—

Remarks: Both hips should be scanned for evaluation of symmetry.

THIGH

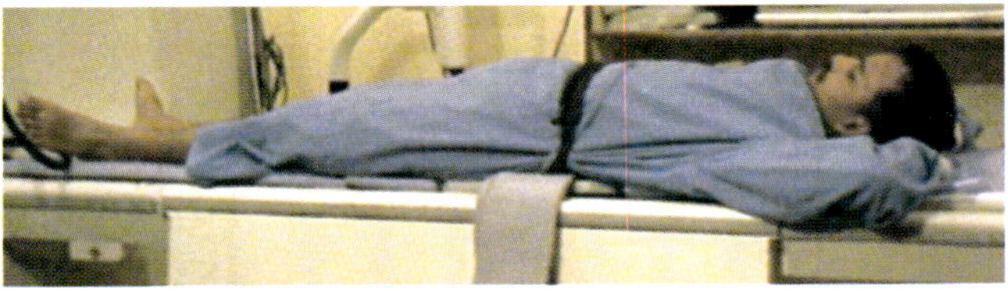

Patient Position- Body coil

- Place the patient supine, feet first.
- Place the thigh in the coil as close as possible to isocenter.
- Position comfort cushions at any pressure points.
- Immobilize the thigh by sliding the small, long cushions.

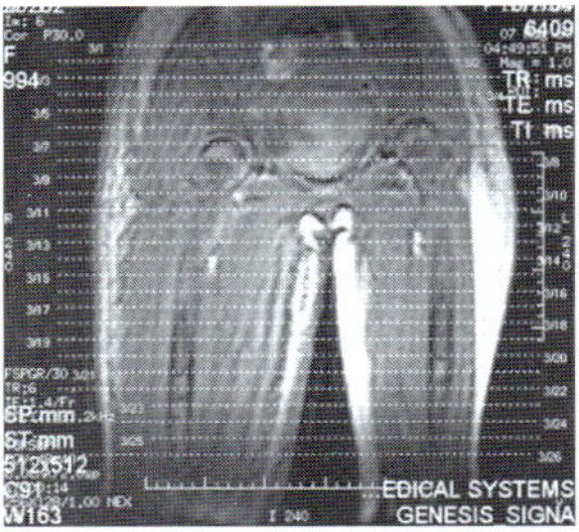

Coronal localizer for axial slices

PROTOCOL: THIGH

Indication

- Visualisation of joint abnormalities
- Visualisation of soft tissue abnormalities

Sequences

Pulse Sequence	Cor T2	Sag T2	Sag STR	O-Axial STIR	O-Axial T2 FSE
TR	4750	5075	5250	4000	5075.0
TE/IR	85	85.0	50/150	80/150	85
ETL	16	16	8	6	16
Bandwidth	20.83	20.83	15.63	15.63	20.83
Nex	3	3	2	3	3
Slice	4	4	4	4	4
Gap	1	1	1	1	1
No. of Slices	20	20	20	16	20
Matrix Freq/Phase	384/256	384/256	256/160	256/192	384/256
FOV	16	16	16	20	16
SNR	100	100	100	100	100
Scan Time	3.52	4.08	3.35	6.32	4.08
Frequency Direction	S/I	A/P	A/P	Unswap	A/P
Auto Center Frequency	Water	Water	Water	Water	Water
Flow Compensation Direction	——	——	——	—	—
Saturation	S,I	S,I	S,I	—	—

Remarks: Both thighs should be scanned for evaluation of symmetry.

KNEE JOINT

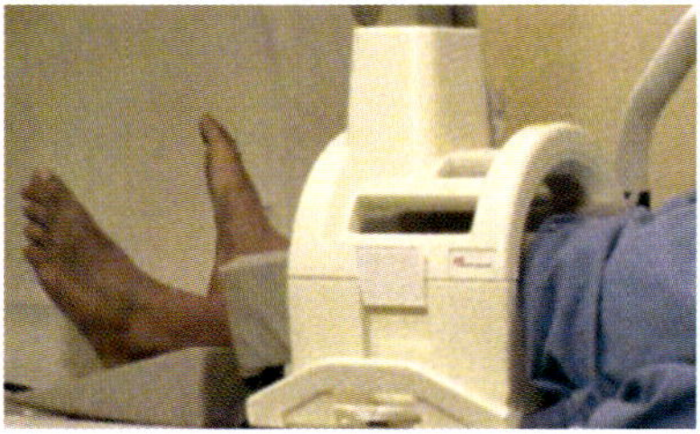

Patient Position-Extremity coil

- Place the patient supine, feet first.
- Place the knee in the bottom half of the coil. Slide the coil bottom along its base until you have the knee as close as possible to isocenter.
- Position comfort cushions at any pressure points with the opposite knee.
- Place cushions under both feet, but don't hyperextend the knee in the coil.
- If you're examining the anterior cruciate ligament, externally rotate the knee per the radiologist's instruction.
- Attach the top half of the coil and lock it in place. Do not pinch any skin between the coil halves.
- Immobilize the knee by sliding the small, long cushions between the knee and the coil.

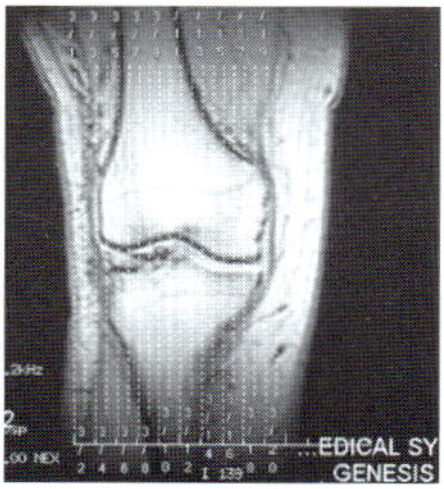

Coronal localizer for sagittal slices

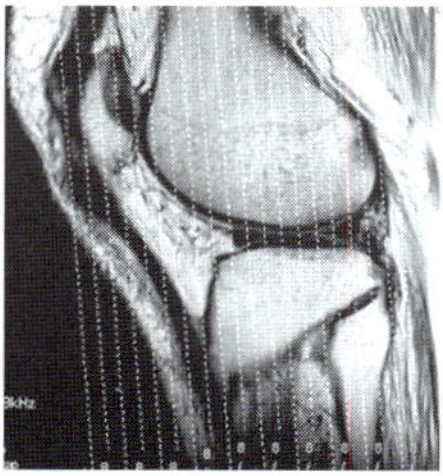

Sagittal localizer for coronal slices

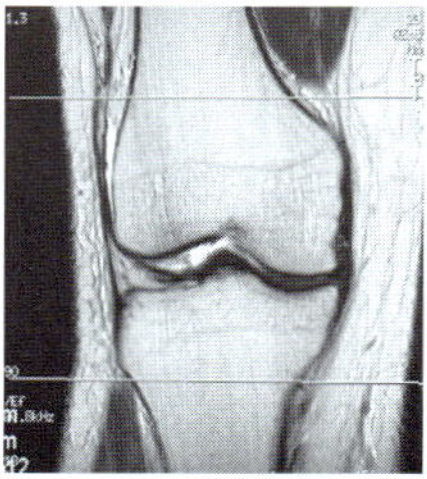

Coronal localizer for axial slices

PROTOCOL: KNEE

Indication

- Assessment of internal derangement of the joint (meniscal tears, cruciate ligament tears, post repair cruciate ligament tears,bursae)
- Evaluation of chondromalacia, patella and patella tracking
- Diagnosis of bone tumors and bony damage within the knee joint
- Almost all other knee disorders can also be visualized

Sequences

Pulse Sequence	Sag T2	Sag T1	Sag STR	Cor T2	Sag T2* GRE	O.COR STIR
TR	5075	550	5250	4750	500	3000
TE/IR	85.0	Min	50/150	85	15.0	68./150
ETL	16	——	8	16	FA:20Degrees	8
Bandwidth	20.83	15.63	15.63	20.83	31.25	15.63
Nex	3	2	2	3	3	2
Slice	4	4	4	4	4	4
Gap	1	1	1	1	1	1.5
No. of Slices	20	20	20	20	20	20
Matrix Freq/Phase	384/256	256/128	256/160	384/256	512/256	256/192
FOV	16	16	16	16	16	16
SNR	100	100	100	100	100	100
Scan Time	4.08	2.25	3.35	3.52	6.28	5.00
Frequency Direction	A/P	R/L	A/P	S/I	S/I	R/L
Auto Center						
Frequency	Water	Water	Water	Water	Water	Water
Flow Compensation Direction	——	——	——	——	——	——
Saturation	S,I	S,I	S,I	S,I	S,I	——

Remarks: Both knees should be scanned for evaluation of symmetry.

TIBIA AND FIBULA

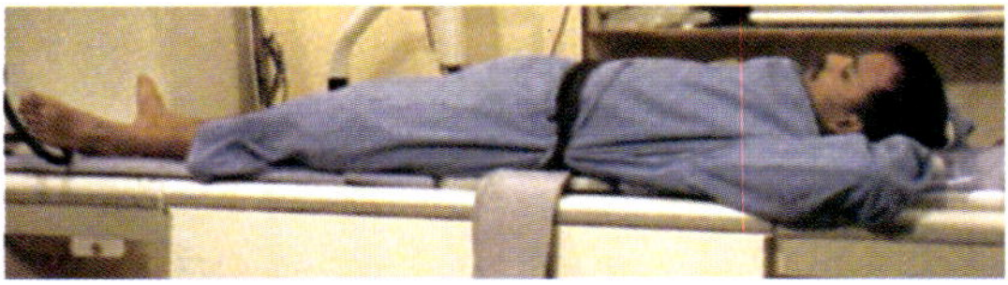

Patient Position- Body coil

- Place the patient supine, feet first.
- Place the leg in the coil as close as possible to isocenter.
- Position comfort cushions at any pressure points.

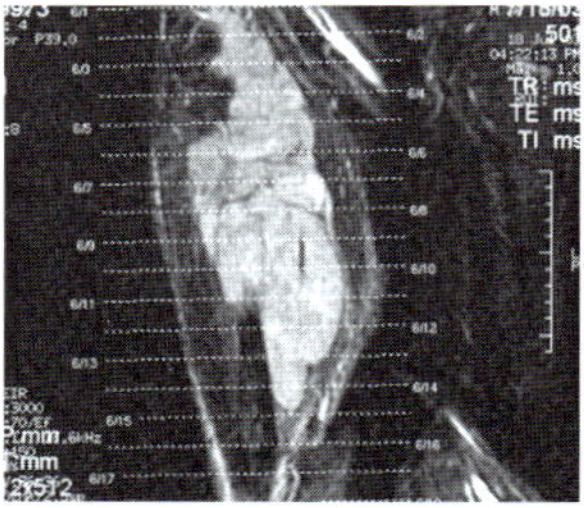

Coronal localizer for axial slices

PROTOCOL: TIBIA AND FIBULA

Indication

- Assessment of suspected or unknown pathology of soft tissue and bone (tumours, infection)

Sequences

Pulse Sequence	O-Cor T1 SE	Cor T2 FSE	O-Ax T1 SE	O-AxT2 FSE	O-Axial STIR	O-Axial T2* GRE
TR	550	4750	650	5575	5325	675
TE/IR	Minimum	85.0	Minimum	85.0	50/150	15.0
ETL	—	16	—	16	8	Flip Angle:20 Deg
Bandwidth	15.63	20.83	20.83	20.83	31.25	31.25
Nex	2	3	3	3	3	3
Slice	4	4	4	4	4	4
Gap	1	1	1	1	1	1
No. of Slices	19	20	20	20	20	20
Matrix Freq/Phase	256/224	384/256	384/256	384/256	320/256	512/256
FOV	16	16	16	16	16	16
SNR	100	100	100	100	100	100
Scan Time	4.05	3.52	5.33	4.32	8.36	8.30
Frequency Direction	S/I	S/I	A/P	A/P	A/P	A/P
Auto Center Frequency	Water	Water	Water	Water	Water	Water
Flow Compensation Direction	—	—	—	—	—	—
Saturation	—	—	S,I	S,I	S,I	S,I

Remarks: Both limbs should be scanned for evaluation of symmetry.

ANKLE

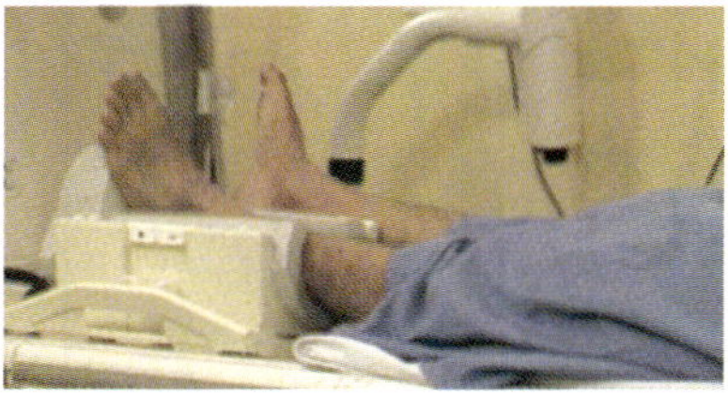

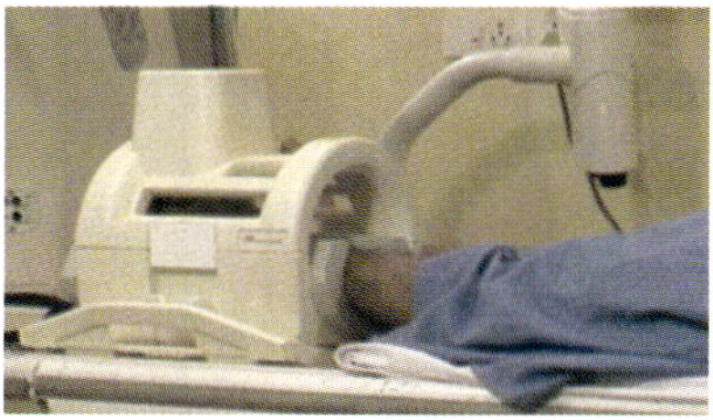

Patient Position- Extremity coil

- Place the patient supine, feet first, with both feet in the coil if possible. If both feet don't fit, place the opposite limb outside the coil and use pads for comfort.
- Centre the anatomy of interest to the coil center.
- Use sponges to elevate the anatomy to isocenter and immobilize with cushions and tape.
- Place cushions at any pressure points to increase comfort and decrease motion.

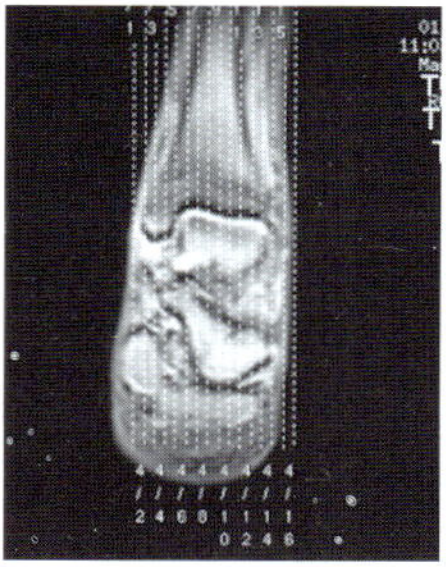

Coronal localizer for

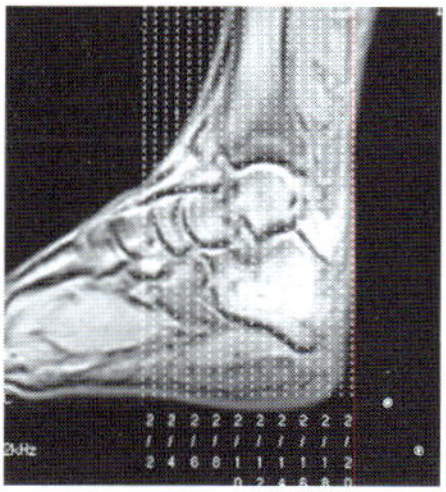

Sagittal localizer for

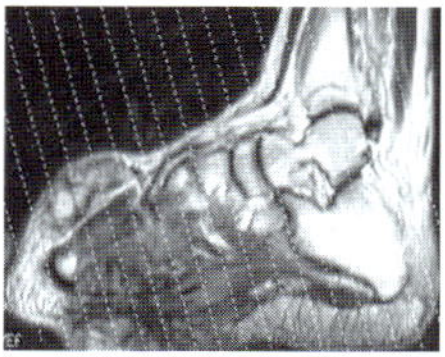

Sagittal localizer for

PROTOCOL: ANKLE

Indication

- Assessment of ankle pain of unknown cause
- Exclusion of osteochondritis dessicans
- Avascular necrosis of the talus
- Visualisation of soft tissue abnormalities
- Assessment of tendonitis (especially posterior tibial)
- Evaluation of achilles tendon rupture or tear
- Evaluation of the ankle joint following trauma
- Possibly useful for evaluation of lateral ligament complex

Sequences

Pulse Sequence	Cor T1 SE	Cor T2 FSE	Cor T2* GRE	Oblique Sag T2	Oblique STIR	Oblique PD
TR	550	5075	500	4300	3000	2400
TE/IR	Minimum	85	15.0	100	50/150	30.0
ETL	—	16	FA-20 Deg	17	8	9
Bandwidth	15.63	20.83	31.25	20.83	15.63	25
Nex	2	3	3	4	2	4
Slice	4	4	4	3	3	3
Gap	1	1	1	0.5	0.5	0.5
No. of Slices	20	20	16	20	20	20
Matrix Freq/Phase	256/224	384/256	512/256	256/192	256/192	256/256
FOV	16	16	16	12	12	12
SNR	102	100	100	100	100	100
Scan Time	4.09	4.08	6.28	3.30	5.00	4.43
Frequency Direction	S/I	A/P	S/I	S/I	S/I	S/I
Auto Center Frequency	Water	Water	Water	Water	Water	Water
Flow Compensation Direction	—	—	—	—	—	—
Saturation	—	a,p	—	—	—	—

VASCULAR IMAGING

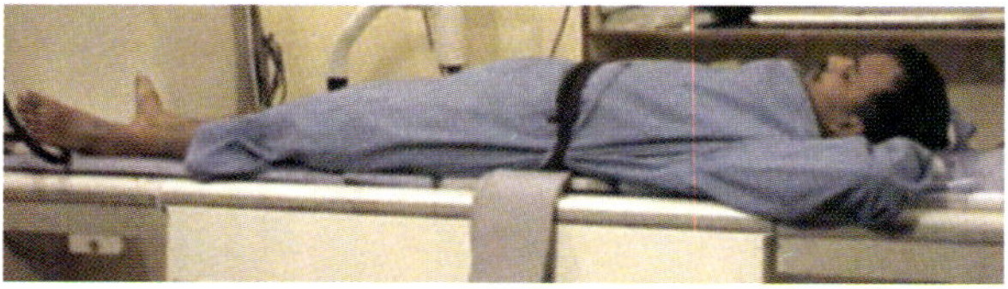

Patient Position: Body coil

- Place the patient supine, feet first.
- Place the leg in the coil as close as possible to isocenter.
- Position comfort cushions at any pressure points.
- Immobilize the leg by sliding the small, long cushions.

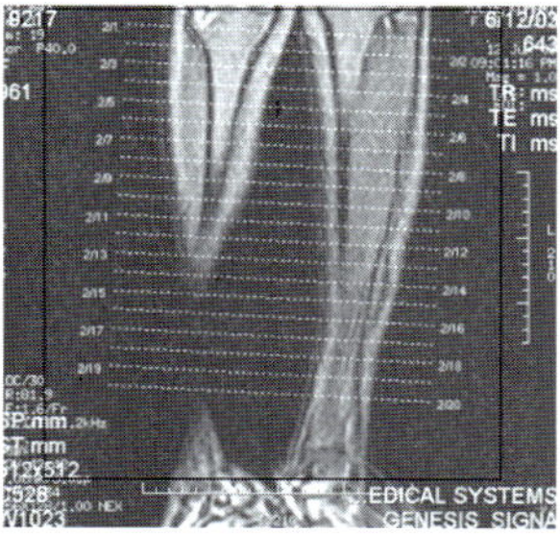

Coronal localizer for axial slices

PROTOCOL: LEG-VASCULAR IMAGING

Indication

- Evaluation of peripheral vascular disease
- Evaluation of normal vasculature (prior to coronary artery by pass surgery to determine the optimal graft site)

Sequences

Pulse Sequence	Gated TOF Angiography Axial	Gated TOF Venography Axial
TR	Minimum	Minimum
TE/IR	Minimum	Minimum
ETL	FA-60 Deg	FA-60 Deg
Bandwidth	15.63	15.63
Nex	1	1
Slice	3	3
Gap	0.5	0.5
No. of Slices	124	124
Matrix Freq/Phase	256/224	256/224
FOV	40	40/.75
SNR	100	100
Scan Time	9.19	9.19
Frequency Direction	R/L	R/L
Auto Center Frequency	Water	Water
Flow Compensation Direction		
Saturation	I	S

MR IMAGES BY ANATOMICAL REGION

ROUTINE IMAGING

- Neuro Imaging
- Neck and spine imaging
- Cardiac imaging
- Abdominal imaging
- Musculoskeletal imaging

VASCULAR IMAGING

SPECIALIZED IMAGING

- Diffusion imaging
- Perfusion imaging
- Functional imaging
- Spectroscopic imaging
- CSF flow
- Steriotactic biopsy

Routine Imaging

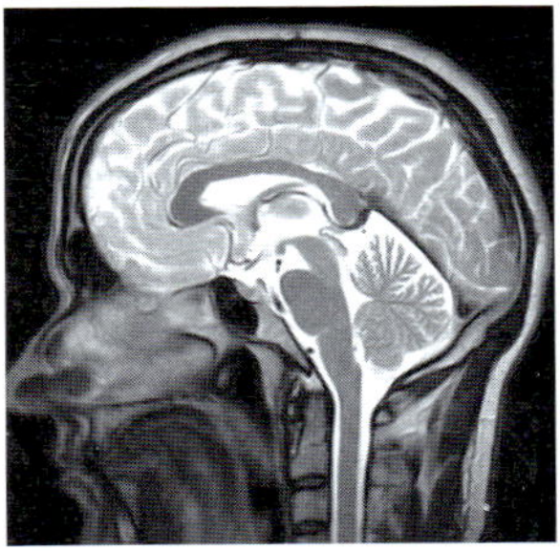

Fast SE T2WI Sagittal-Brain

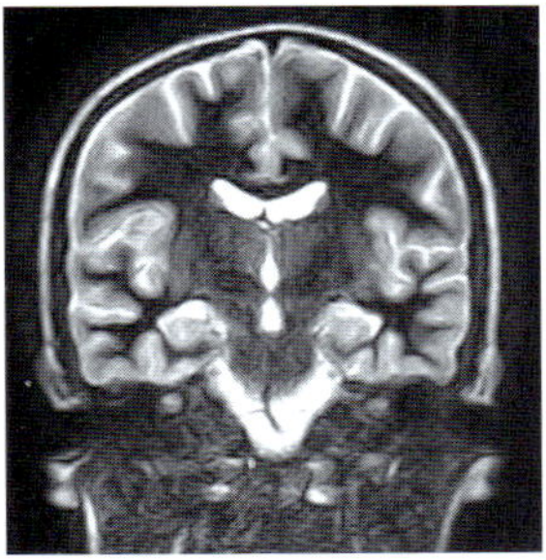

Fast SE T2WI Coronal-Brain

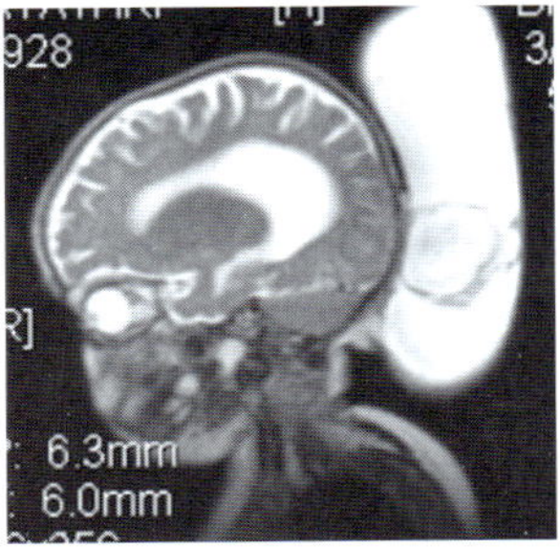

FSE T2WI Sagittal-Brain

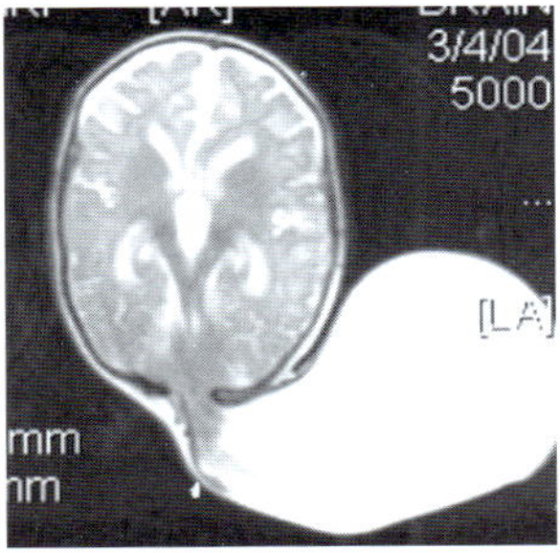

FSE T2W Axial-Brain

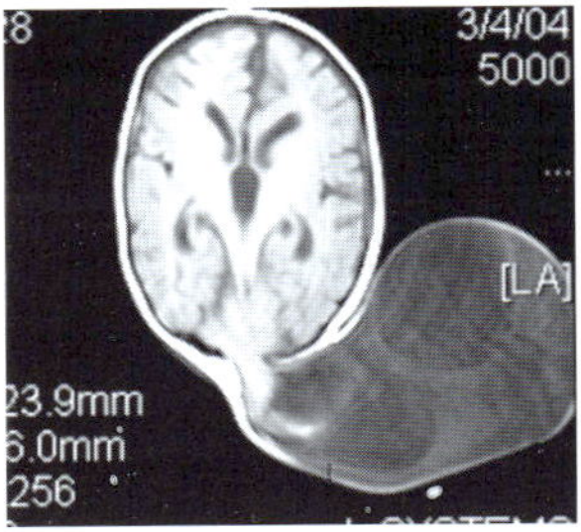

FSE T1WI Axial-Brain

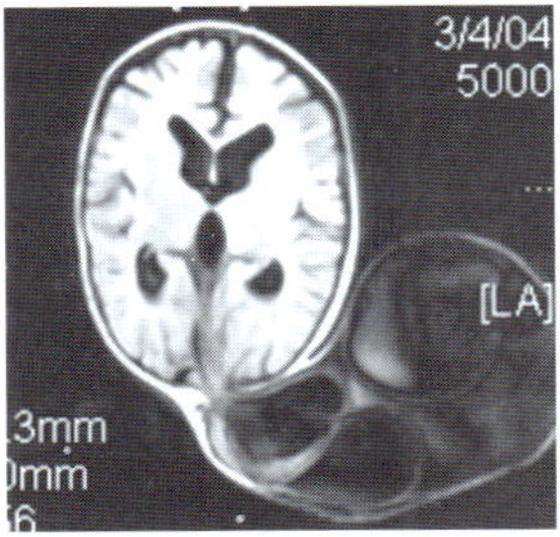

FLAIR Axial-Brain

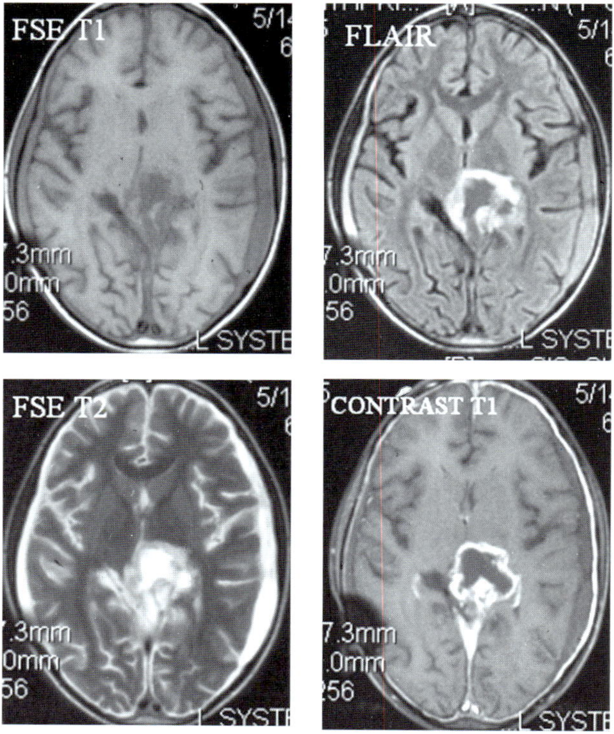

Postoperative case of pilocytic astrocytoma of brainstem extending into left thalamus with b/l subdural haemorrhage

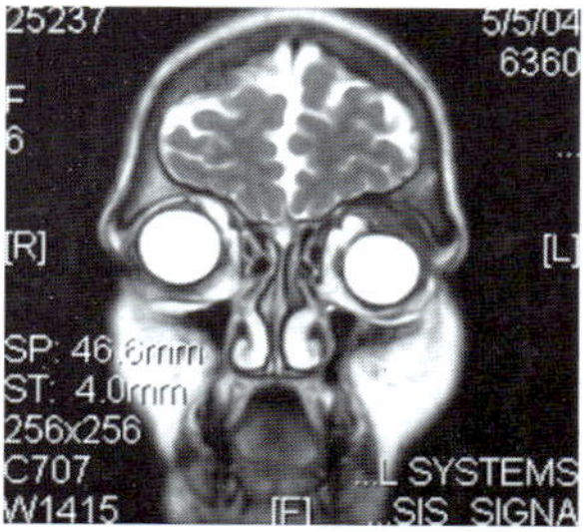

FSE T2WI coronal-orbit

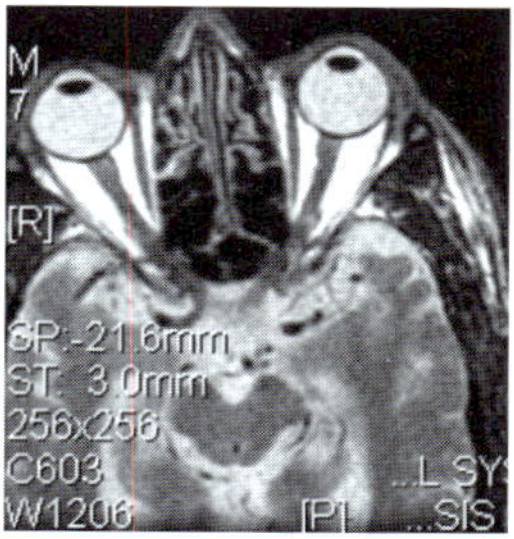

FSE T2 WI axial orbit

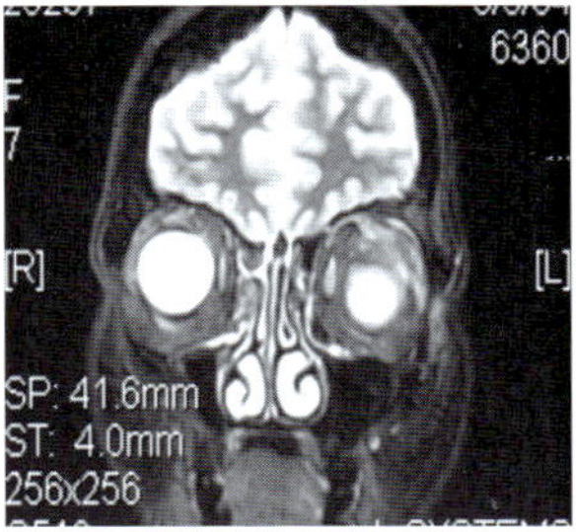

STIR coronal -orbit

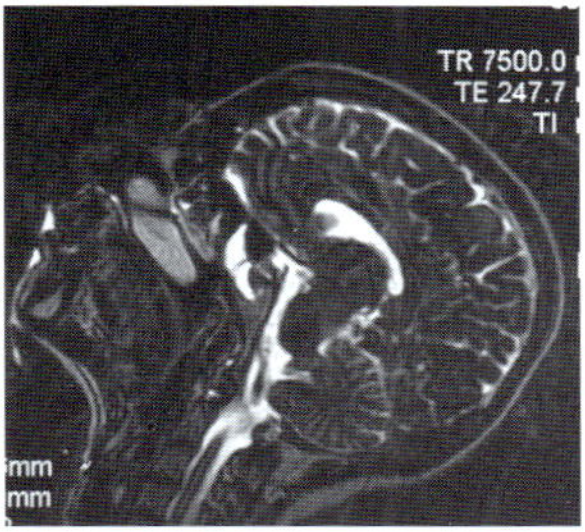

Heavily FSE T2 WI sagittal prone-CSF rhinorrhea

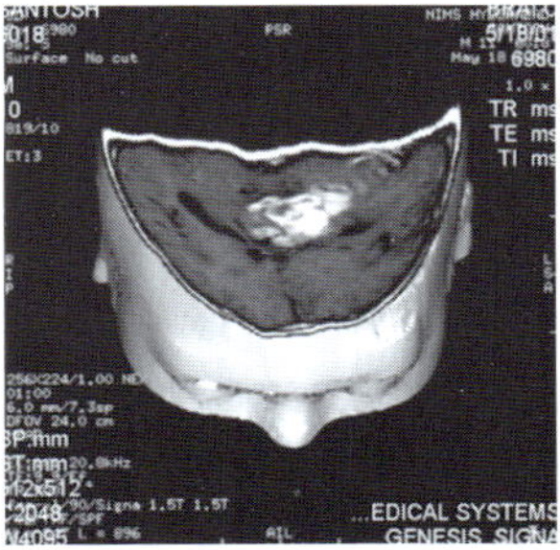

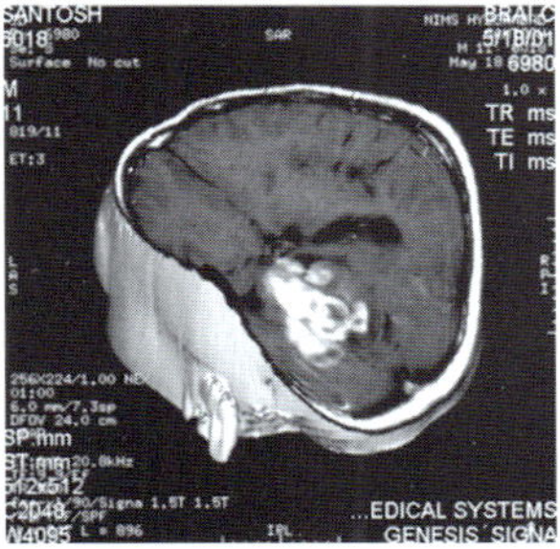

3D reconstruction

Neck and Spine Imaging

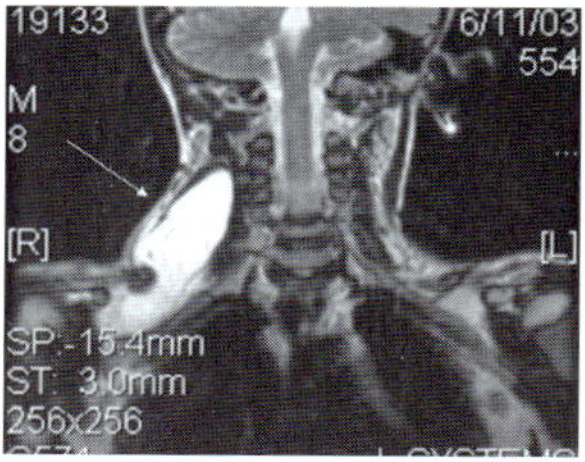

FSE T2WI coronal neck plexiform neurofibroma

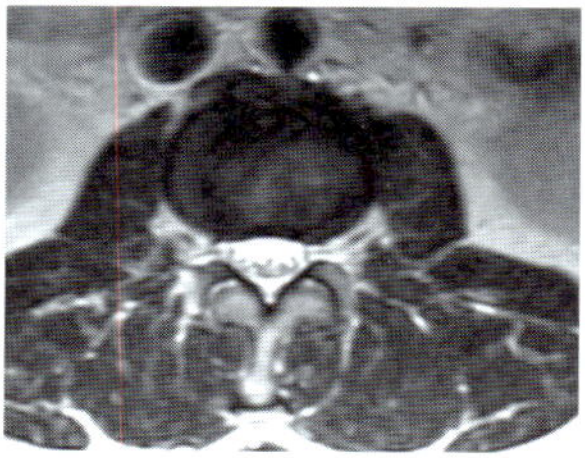

FSE T2WI axial -lumbar disc

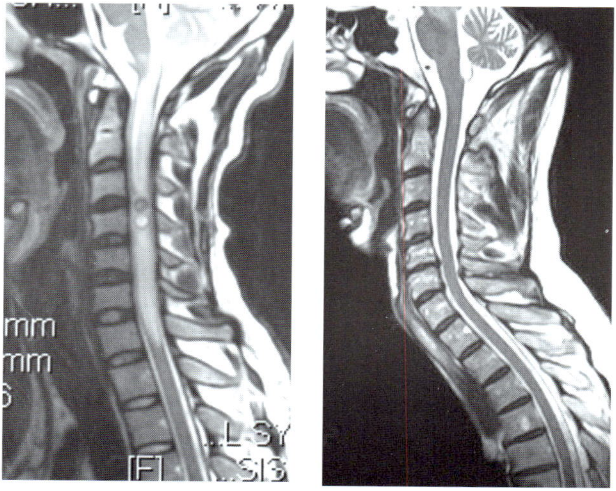

FSE T2WI sagittal -cervical spine

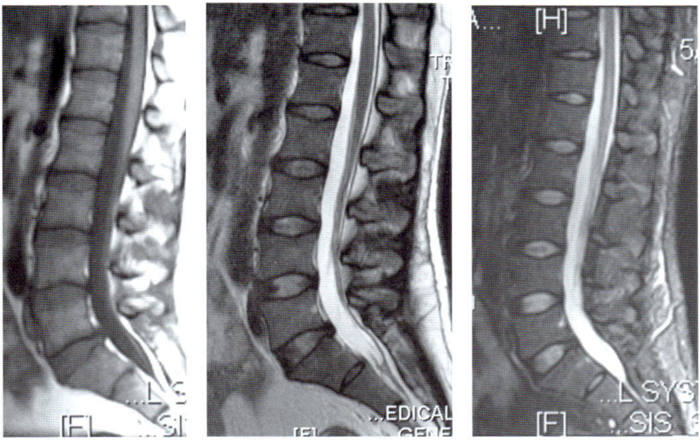

FSE T1W I FSE T2WI STIR

Lumbar spine-sagittal images

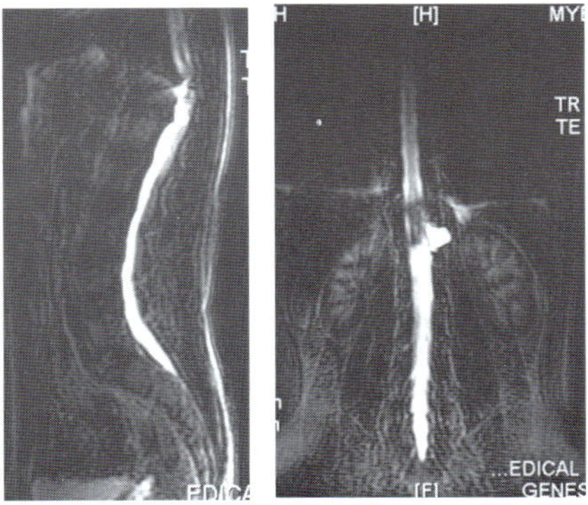

Myelograms of DL spine

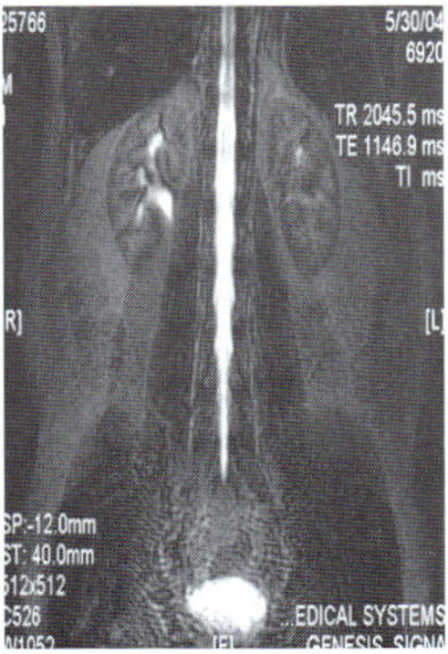

Myelogram of L-spine

Cardiac Imaging

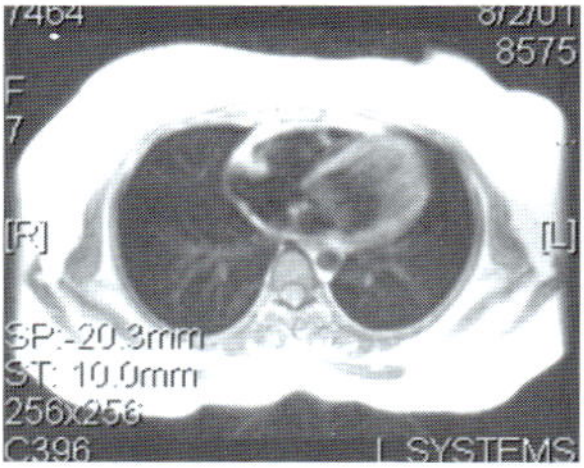

SE T1W axial -heart with ECG gating

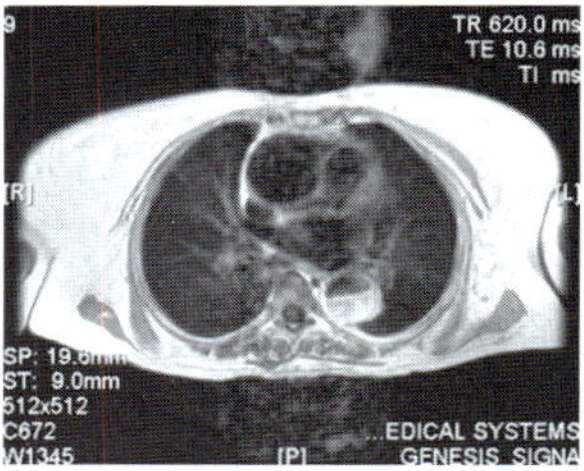

SE T1W axial -heart Dissection of descending aorta

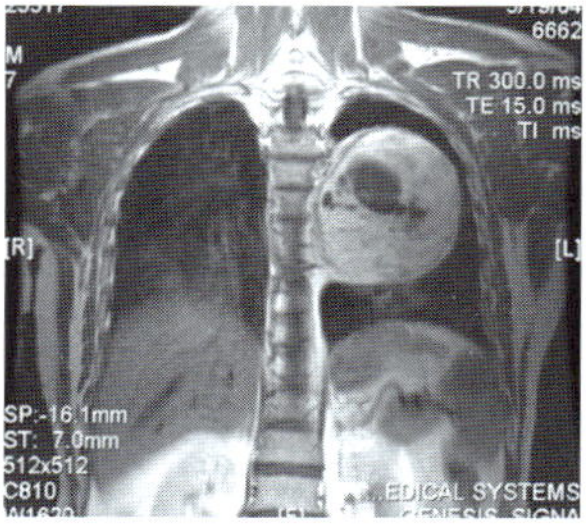

Cornal SE T1WI -chest

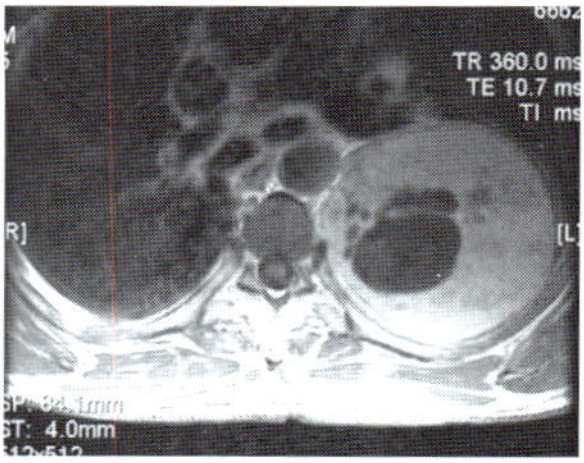

Axial SE T1WI-chest

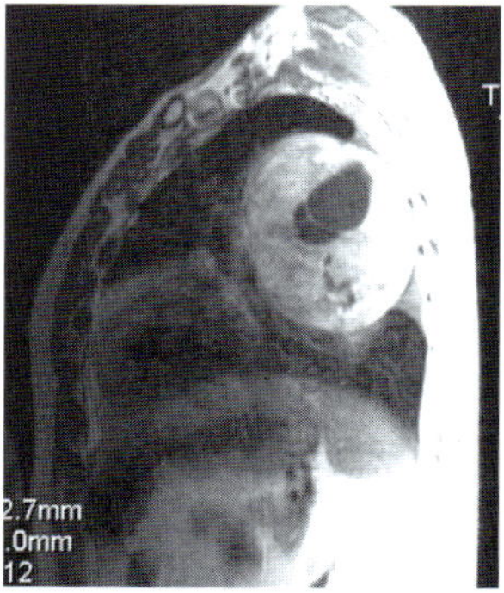

Sagittal SE T1WI -chest

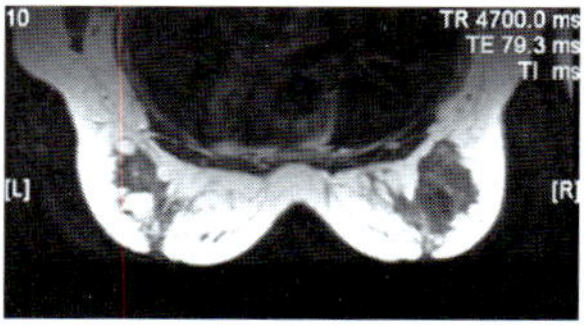

Axial FSE T2W I-breast

Abdominal Imaging

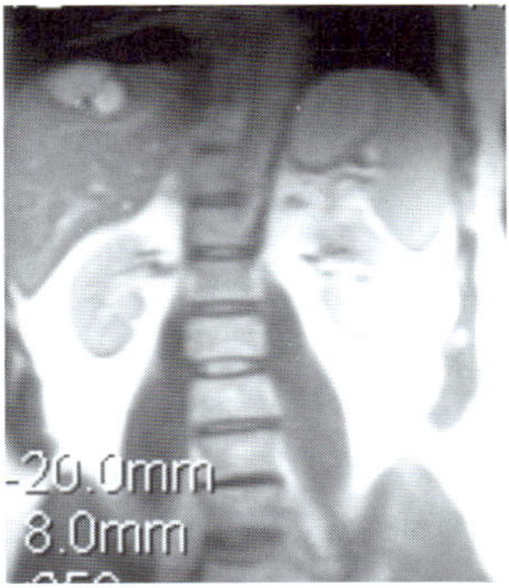

Coronal fast SPGR -abdomen

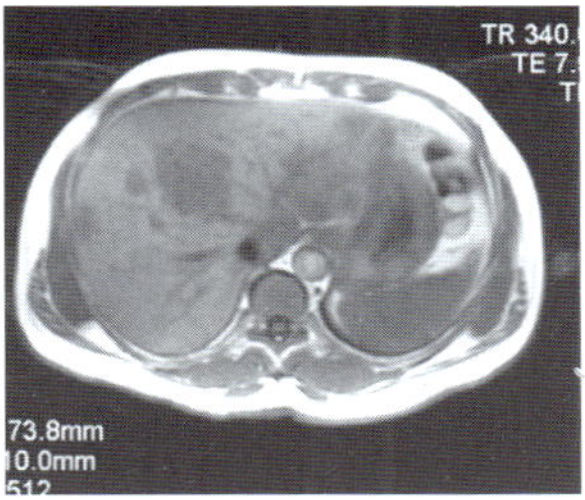

Axial SE T1WI- abdomen

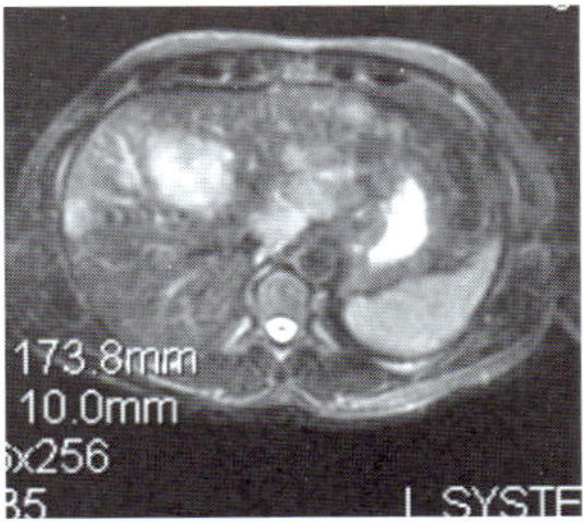

Axial STIR -abdomen

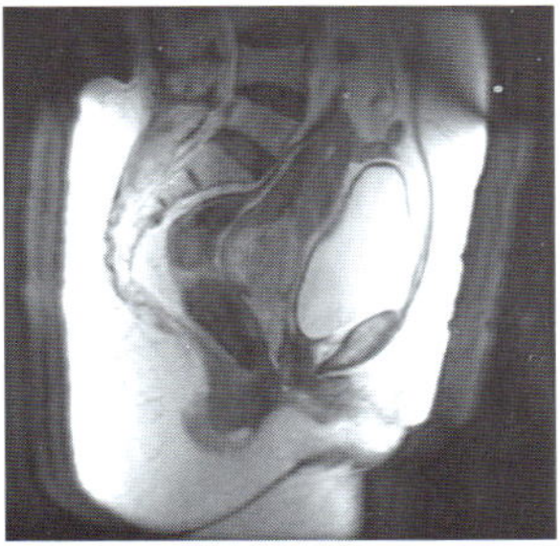

Ca cervix along with fibroid uterus
sagittal FSE T2WI-pelvis

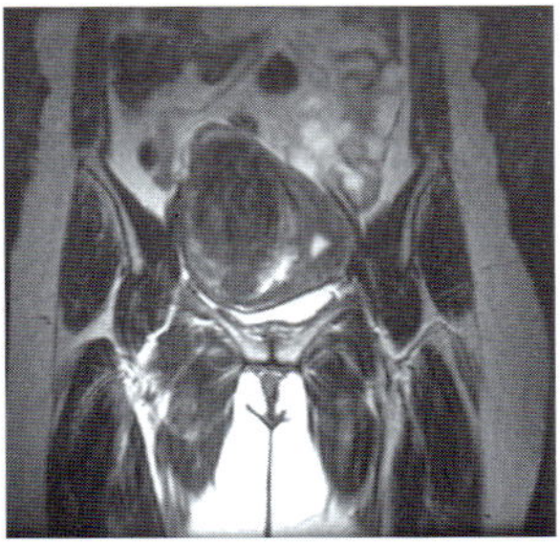

Coronal FSE T2WI -pelvis
fibroid uterus

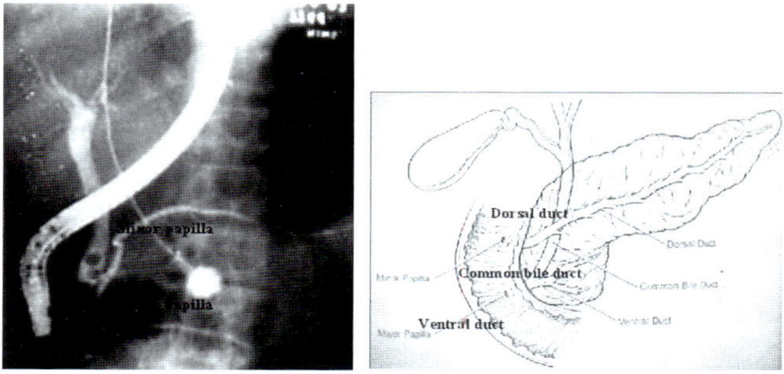

ERCP- lower CBD stone

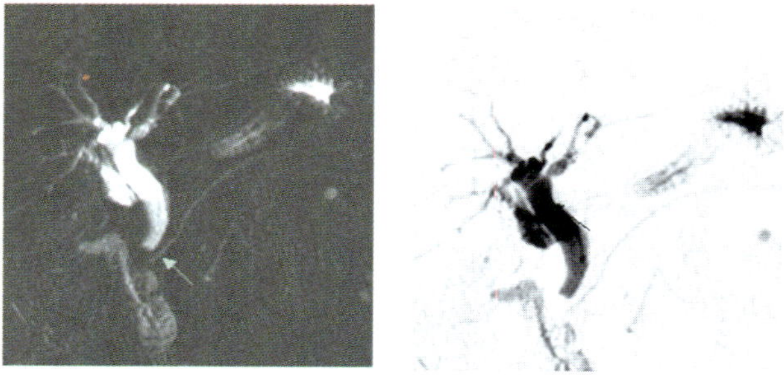

MRCP-postcholecystectomy CBD calculus

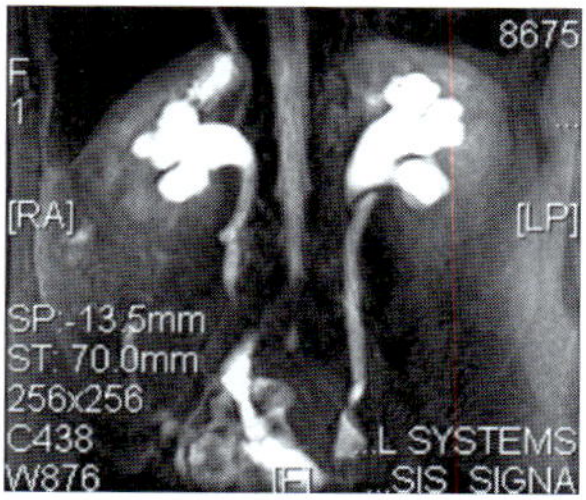

MR urography

Musculoskeletal Imaging

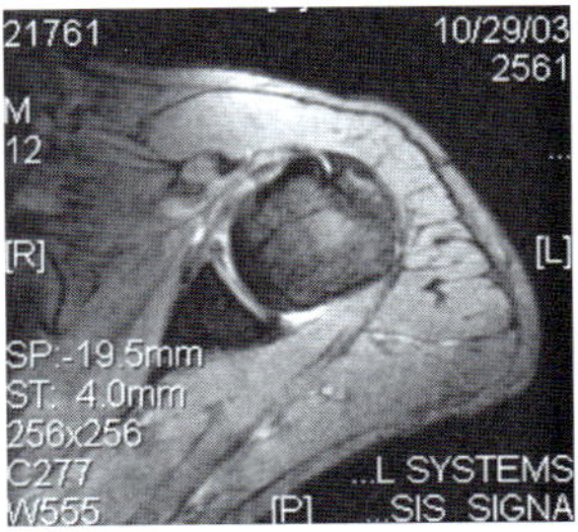

O-axial gradient shoulder

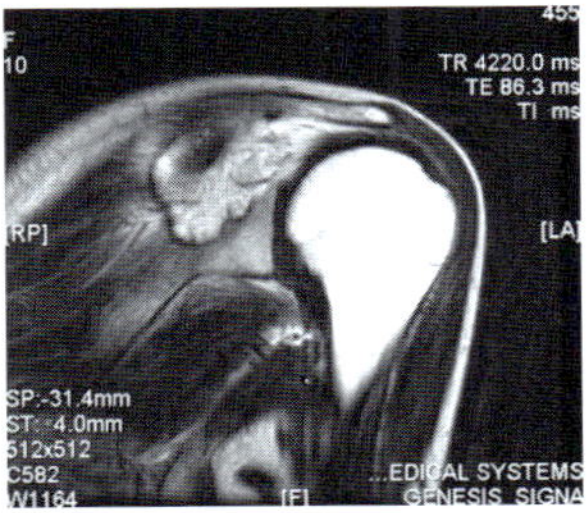

O-coronal FSE T2WI - shoulder

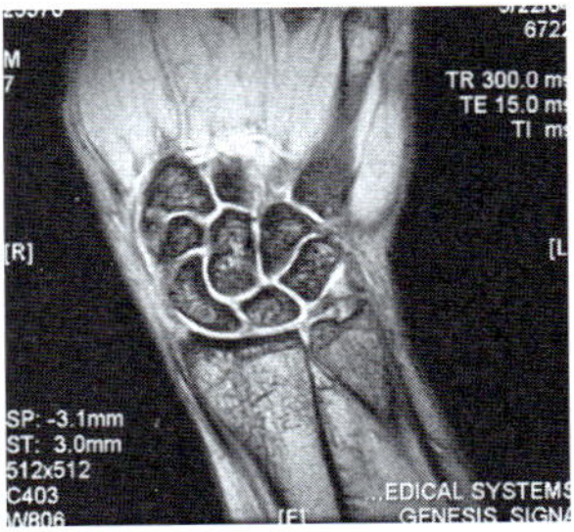

Gradient coronal -hand

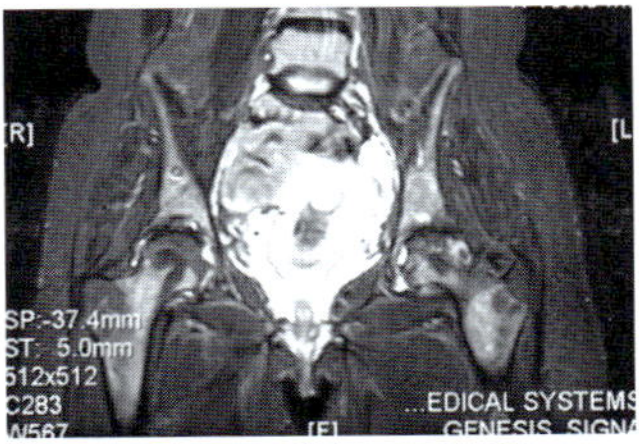

Coronal stir -both hip joints juvenile chronic arthritis with involvement of b/l hip joints

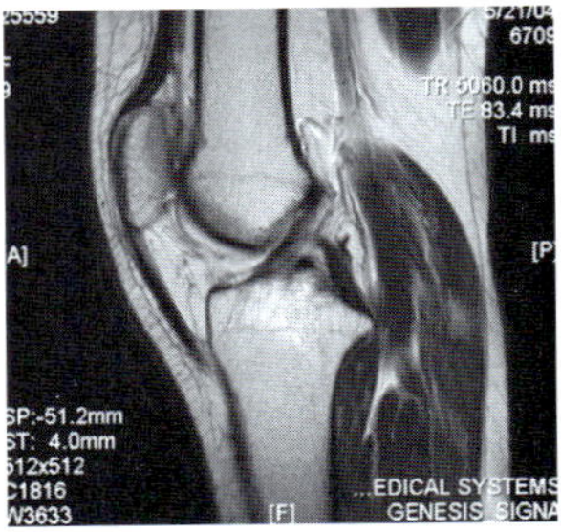

FSE T2WI sagittal -knee joint

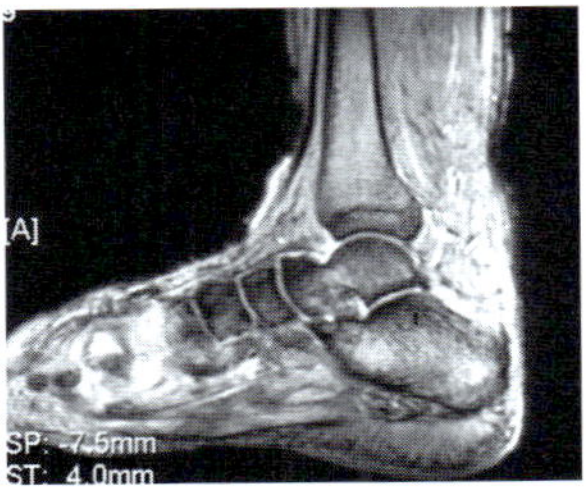

Gradient sagittal -ankle joint diabetic foot

VASCULAR IMAGING

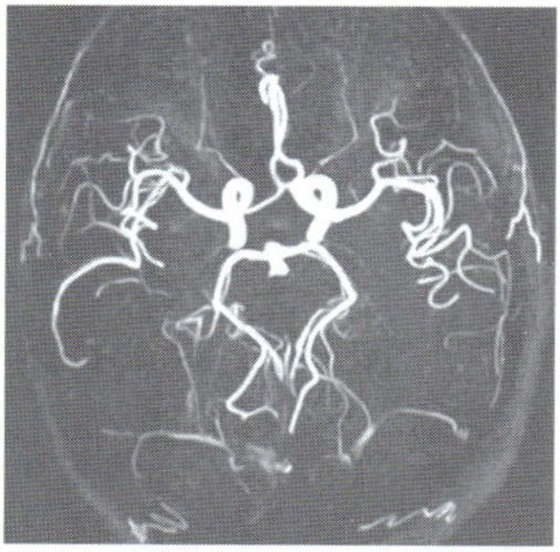

TOF acquisition of circle of Willis

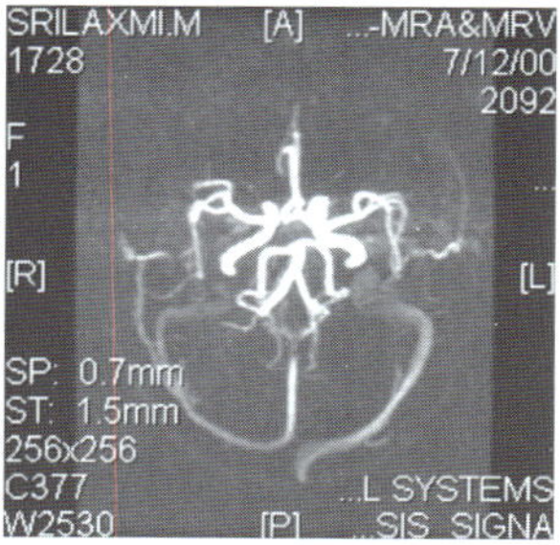

3D PC intracranial angio

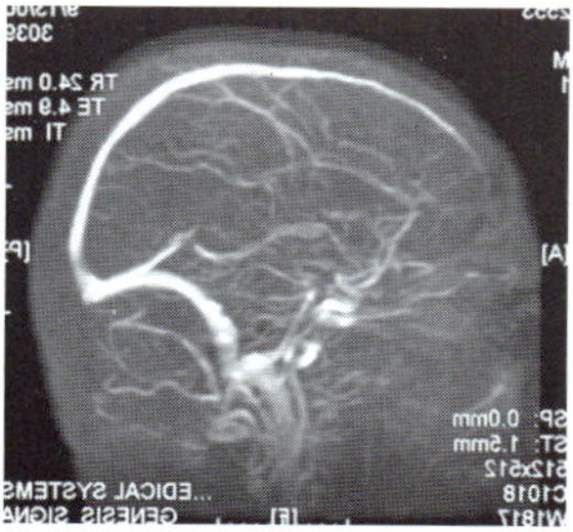

2D TOF-MRV

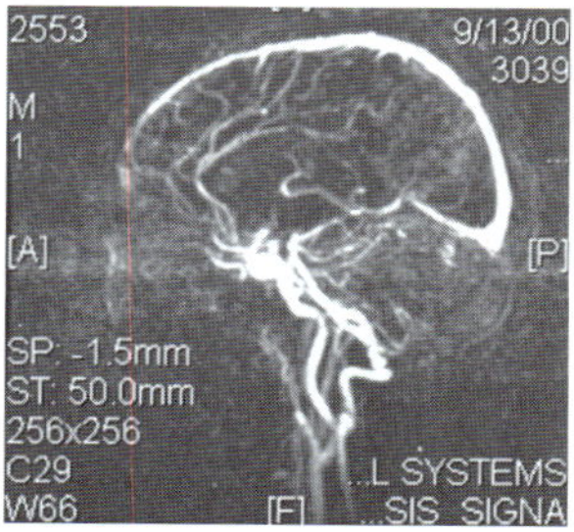

SAG-2D PC-MRV

Normal MRV

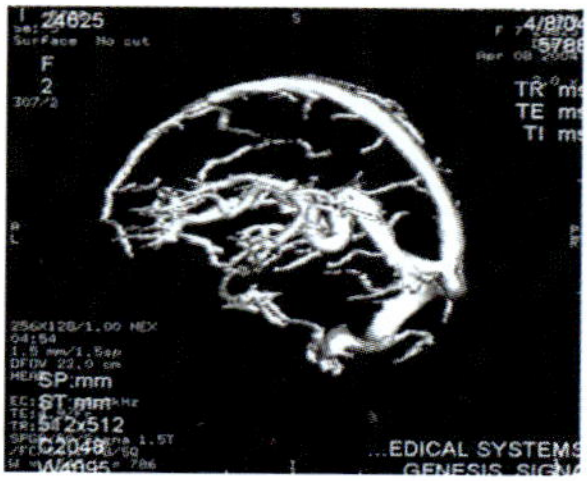

SSD-MRV

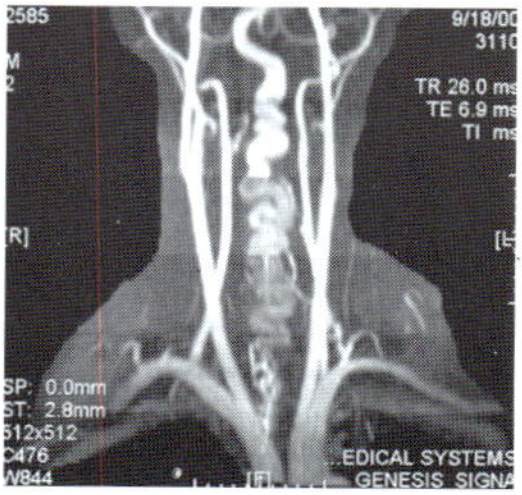

2DTof-motsa (6 slab) acquisition MRA extracranial vessels with spinal AVM

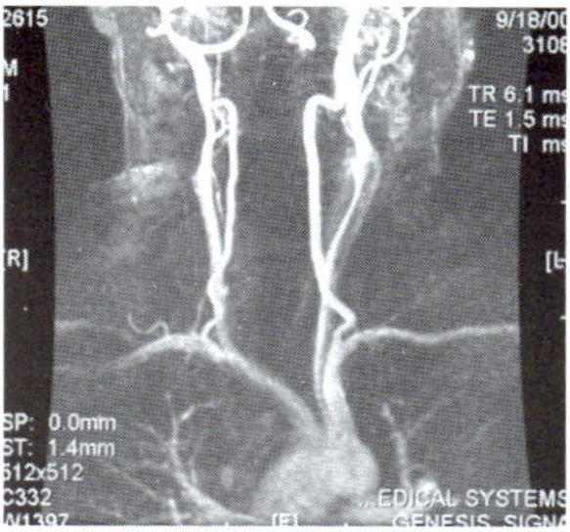

Contrast enhanced MRA
of neck vessels

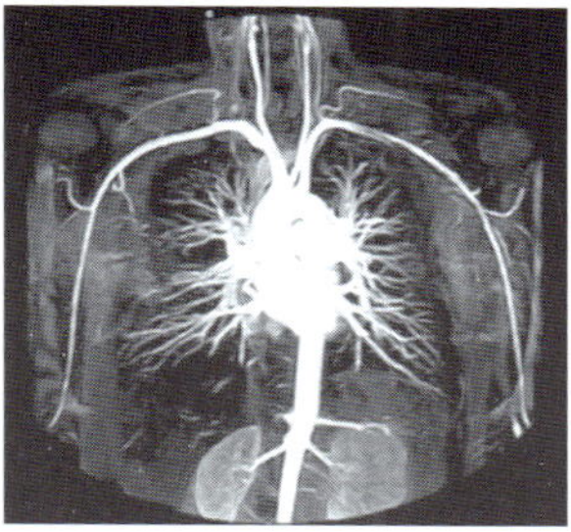

Contrast enhanced angiography
of aorta and its branches

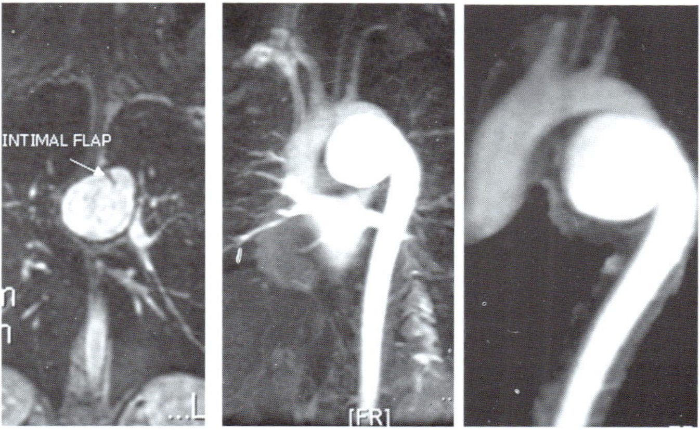

Post-traumatic aortic aneurysm
39 years/male, H/O RTA 10-yr back. Incidentally detected aortic
aneurysm in 1999 at UGI endoscopy

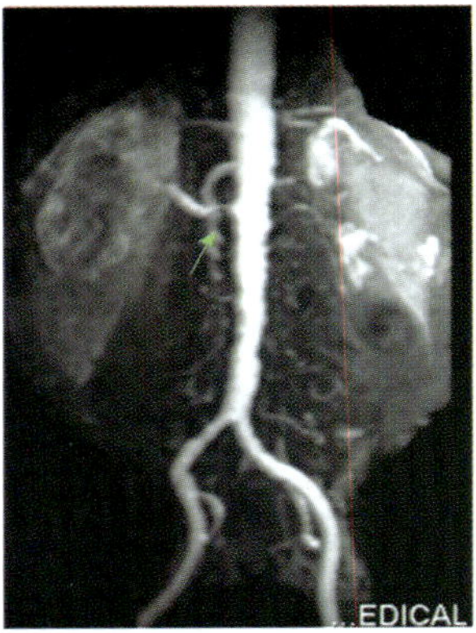

RT. Renal artery stenosis

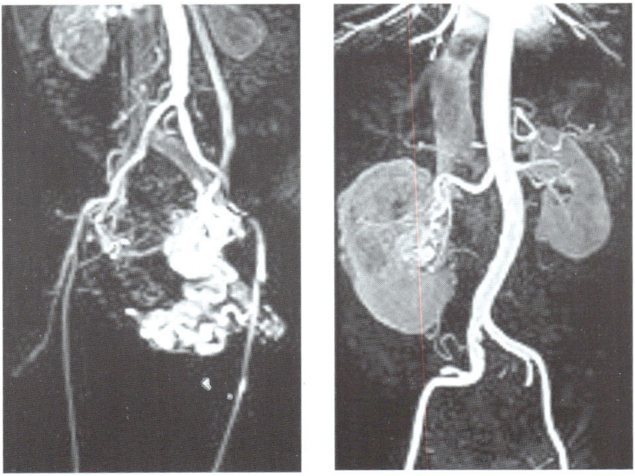

Contrast enhanced abdominal angiogram

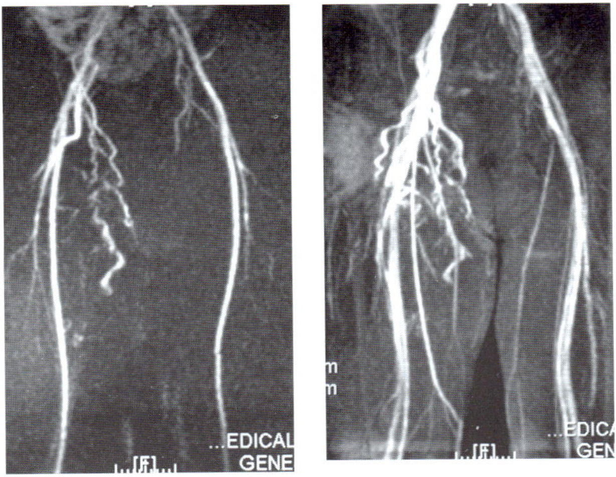

AVM Thigh
30 Y/M, follow-up case of AVM RT thigh—post-embolisation

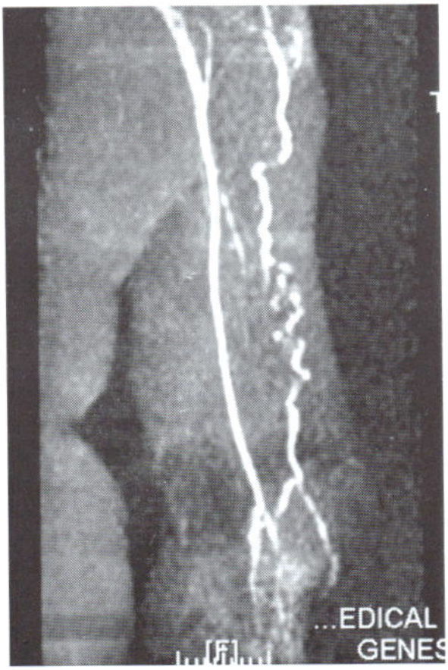

TOF acquisition with ECG gating of
ARM -without contrast

SPECIALIZED IMAGING

Diffusion Imaging

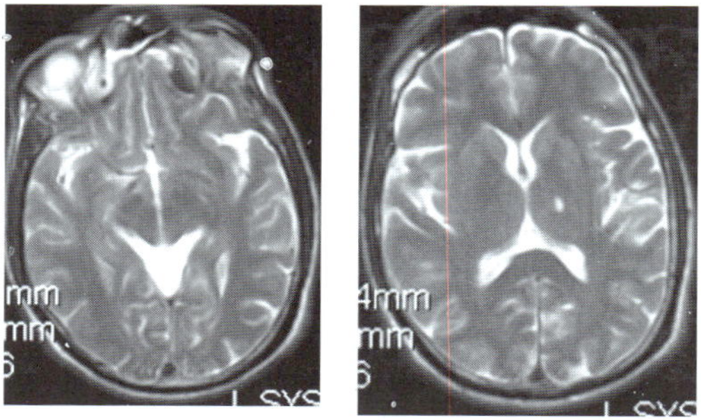

T2WI

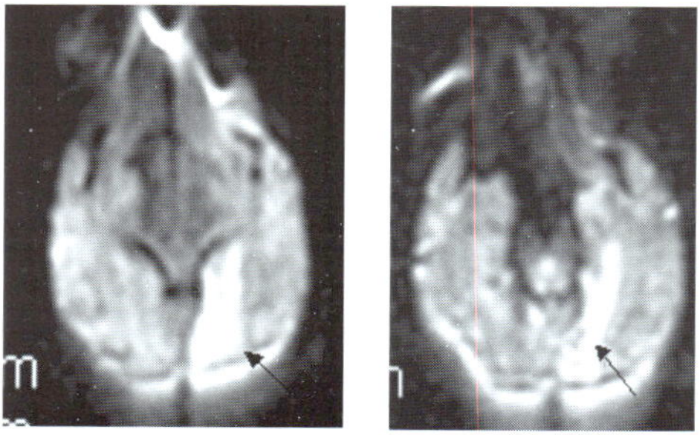

DWI

Acute PCA territory stroke

42 M, with suspected posterior circulation stroke

Perfusion Imaging

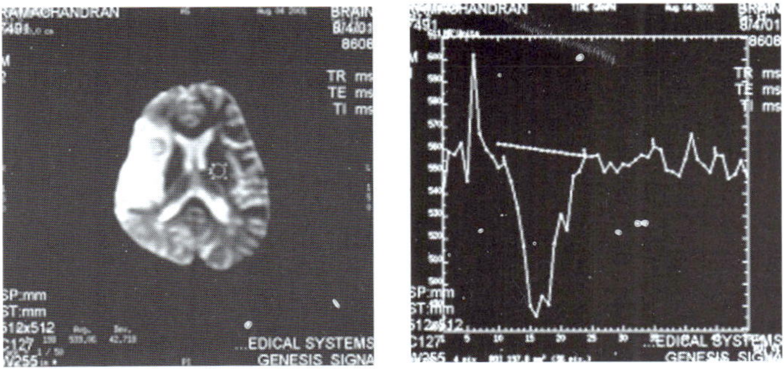

Normal

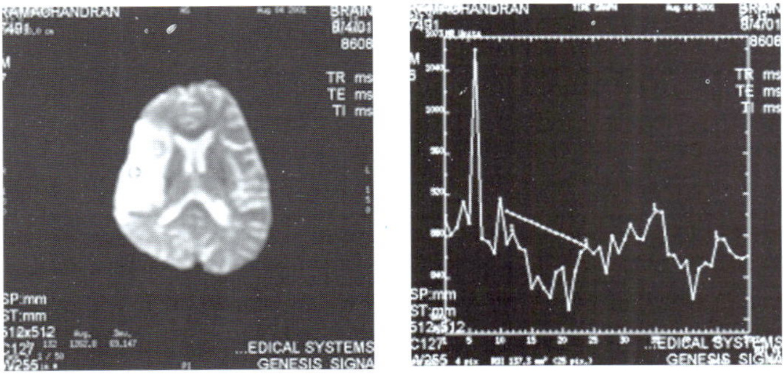

Abnormal

Functional Imaging

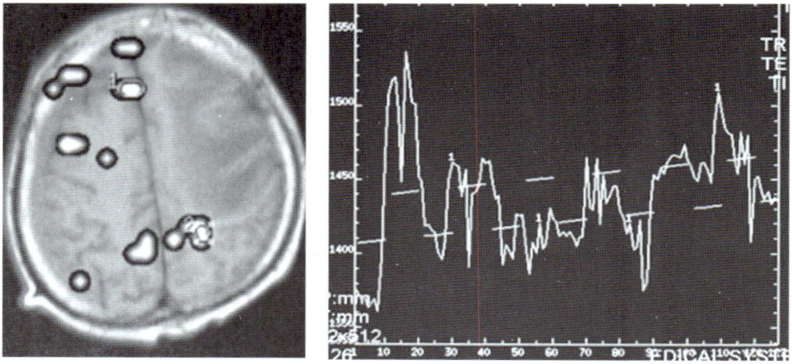

Localisation of speech cortex
young adult with glioma. lt parietal cortex
functional MRI-preop

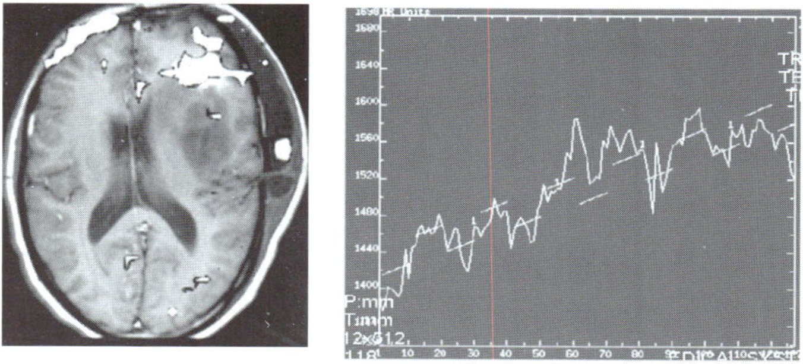

Localisation of speech cortex
functional MR - postop

Spectroscopic Imaging

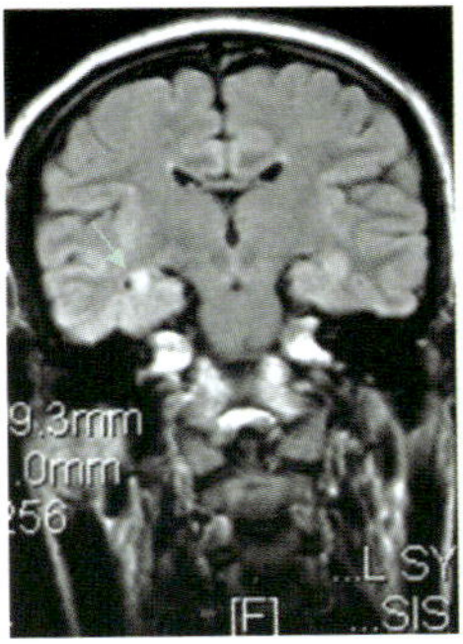

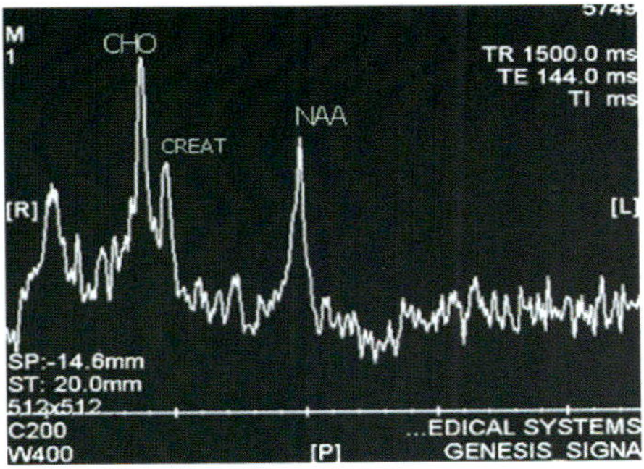

Cor FSEIR MRS

Mesial temporal sclerosis

22 M, H/O seizures since 5-yr on antiepileptic medication

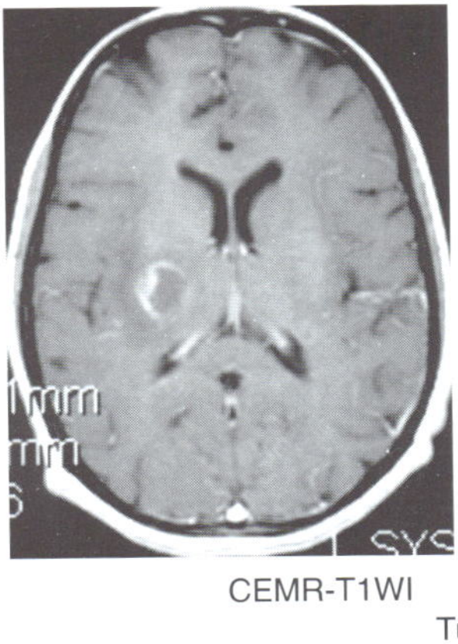

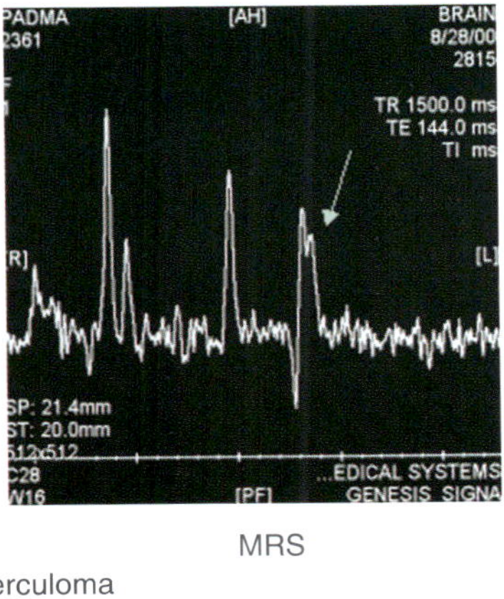

CEMR-T1WI MRS

Tuberculoma

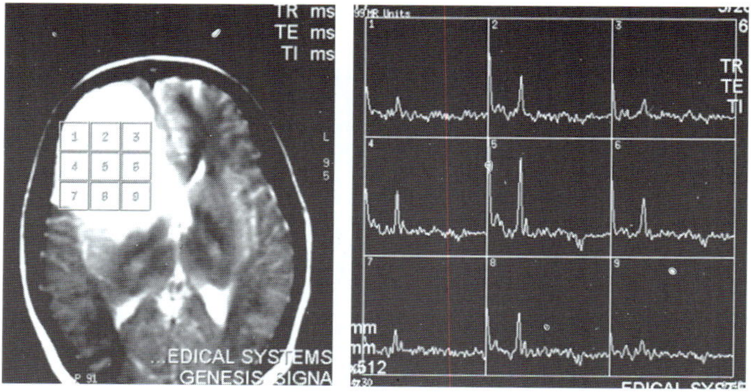

Multi voxel-spectroscopy

CSF Flow

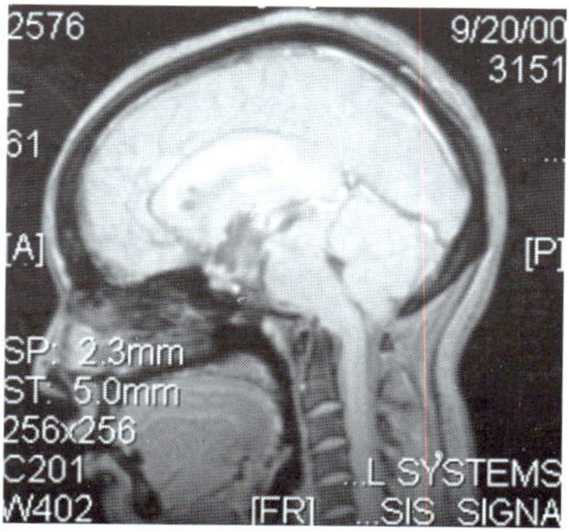

CSF flow

Steriotactic Biopsy

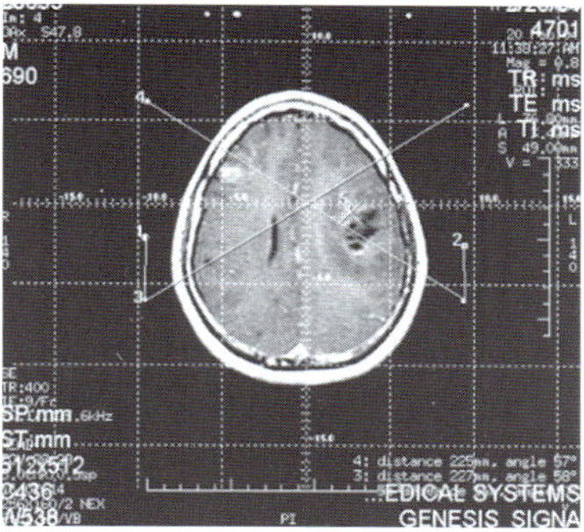

Steriotaxic biopsy

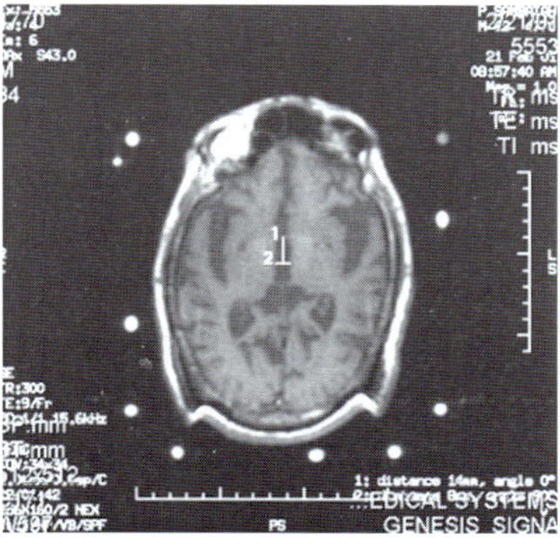

Deep brain stimulation (DBS)

Abbreviations

2DFT	:	Two-Dimensional Fourier Transformation
3-D	:	Three Dimensional
A	:	Anterior
AAA	:	Abdominal Aortic Aneurysm
ACA	:	Anterior Cerebral Artery
ACM	:	Arnold-Chiari Malformation
ACQ	:	Acquisition
A/P	:	Anterior/Posterior
AP	:	Anterioposterior
AP	:	Array Processor
AVM	:	Arteriovenous Malformation
AVN	:	Avascular Necrosis
BOLD	:	Blood Oxygenation Level Dependent
CAD	:	Coronary Artery Disease
CBD	:	Common Bile Duct
CBF	:	Cerebral Blood Flow
CDJ	:	Cervico Dorsal Spine Junction
CF	:	Center Frequency
CHA	:	Common Hepatic Artery

Chem Sat	:	Chemical Shift Saturation
CHO	:	Choline
CM	:	Contrast Medium
CN Ratio	:	Contrast to Noise Ratio
CNS	:	Central Nervous System
COPD	:	Chronic Obstructive Pulmonary Disease
CR	:	Creatinine
CSE	:	Conventional Spin Echo
CSF	:	Cerebro Spinal Fluid
CSVT	:	Cortical Sinus Venous Thrombosis
CVA	:	Cerebro Vascular Accident
CVJ	:	Cranio Vertebral Junction
CXR	:	Chest X-Ray
Db	:	Decibels
DICOM	:	Digital Imaging and Communications in Medicine
DLJ	:	Dorso Lumbar Junction
DM	:	Diabetes Mellitus
DSA	:	Digital Subtraction Angiography
DVT	:	Deep Vein Thrombosis
EAM	:	External Auditory Meatus
ECG	:	Electro Cardiogram Gating
EDH	:	Extra Dural Hematoma
EHBO	:	Extra Hepatic Biliary Obstruction
EPI	:	Echo Planar Imaging
ETL	:	Echo Train Length
FA	:	Flip Angle

FAT	:	Fat
FC	:	Flow Compensation
FDD	:	Floppy Disk Drive
F/F	:	Feet First
FFE	:	Fast Field Echo
FID	:	Free Induction Decay
FOV	:	Field of View
FSE	:	Fast Spin Echo
GA	:	General Anaesthesia
GB	:	Gall Bladder
gd	:	gadolinium
GIT	:	Genito Intestinal Tract
GRASS	:	Gradient Recalled Acquisition the Steady State
GRE	:	Gradient Recalled Echo
HASTE	:	Half Fourier Acquisition Single Shot Turbo Spin Echo
HDD	:	Hard Disk Drive
H/F	:	Head First
HNR	:	Head and Neck Region
HTN	:	Hyper Tension
I	:	Inferior
IAC	:	Internal Auditory Canal
IAM	:	Internal Auditory Meatus
ICA	:	Internal Carotid Artery
IHBC	:	Intra Hepatic Biliary Canaliculi
IHBD	:	Intra Hepatic Biliary Dilatation

IHBO	:	Intra Hepatic Biliary Obstruction
IOML	:	Infra Orbito Meatal Line
IRFSE	:	Inversion Recovery Fast Spin Echo
IV	:	Intravenous
IVC	:	Inferior Vena Cava
IVD	:	Inter Vertebral Disc
IVU	:	Intra Venous Urogram
L	:	Left
LAT	:	Lateral
LN	:	Lymph Node
LSJ	:	Lumbo Sacral Spine Junction
MCA	:	Middle Cerebral Artery
ME	:	Multi Echo
Min-	:	Minimum
Min-IP	:	Minimum Intensity Projection
MIP	:	Maximal Intensity Projection
mm	:	millimeter
MOD	:	Magneto Optical Disc
MOTSA	:	Multiple Overlapping Thin Section Angiography
MPR	:	Multi Planar Reconstruction
MR	:	Magnetic Resonance
MRCP	:	Magnetic Resonance Cholangio Pancreotography
MRI	:	Magnetic Resonance Imaging
MRS	:	MR Spectroscopy
MRU	:	Magnetic Resonance Urography

MS	:	Milli Seconds
MS	:	Multiple Sclerosis
MSK	:	Musculo Skeletal
MTC	:	Magnetization Transfer Contrast
MV	:	Multi Voxel
NAA	:	N-Acetylaspartate
Nex	:	Number of Excitations
NMR	:	Nuclear Magnetic Resonance
NMV	:	Net Magnetization Vector
NP	:	Number of Phase Encodings
NPW	:	No. Phase Wrap
NS	:	Number of Slice Encodings
NSA	:	Number of Signal Averaged
OC	:	Operators Console
OML	:	Orbito Meatal Line
OPLL	:	Ossification of Posterior Longitudinal Ligament
P	:	Posterior
PC	:	Phase Contrast
PCA	:	Phase Contrast Angiography
PCA	:	Posterior Cerebral Artery
PCA	:	Posterior Communicating Artery
PD	:	Proton Density
PE	:	Pulmonary Embolism
Pe-gating	:	Peripheral Gating
PIVD	:	Protruded Inter Vertebral Disk
PNS	:	Para Nasal Sinus

PO	:	Postoperative
PPM	:	Parts Per Million
Pr Inj.	:	Pressure Injector
PRESS	:	Point Resolved Spectroscopy
Probe	:	Proton Brain Examination
PS	:	Partial-Saturation
PS	:	Pulse Sequence
PSD	:	Phase Sensitive Detection
PUJ	:	Pelvi Ureteric Junction
R	:	Right
RAT	:	Renal Artery Thrombosis
RC	:	Respiratory Compensation
RCBV	:	Regional Cerebral Blood Volume
RCC	:	Renal Cell Carcinoma
Reconstr	:	Reconstruction
Ref	:	Reference
REST	:	Regional Saturation Technique
RF	:	Radio Frequency
R/L	:	Right/Left
R/O	:	Rule Out
ROI	:	Region of Interest
RR	:	R to R Interval
RT	:	Rectangular Field of View
RVT	:	Renal Vein Thrombosis
S	:	Superior
SAH	:	Subarachnoid Hemorrhage
SAR	:	Specific Absorption Rate

SAT	:	Pre Saturation Pulse
SCJ	:	Sterno Clavicular Joint
SCM	:	System Control Module
SDH	:	Sub Dural Hematoma
SE	:	Spin-Echo Pulse Sequence
Sec.	:	Second
S/I	:	Superior/Inferior
SL No.	:	Slice Number
SL Thick	:	Slice Thickness
SNR	:	Signal-to-Noise Ratio
SOL	:	Space Occupying Lesion
SP	:	Spine
SPGR	:	Spoiled GRASS
SR	:	Saturation-Recovery Pulse Sequence
SS FP	:	Steady State Free Precession
SS FSE	:	Signal Shot Fast Spin Echo
SSD	:	Shaded Surface Display
STIR	:	Short TI Inversion Recovery Pulse Sequence
SV	:	Single Voxel
SVC	:	Superior Vena Cava
T1	:	Longitudinal Relaxation Time
T2	:	Transverse Relaxation Time
T2*	:	The Time Constant of the FID Signal
TB	:	Temporal Bone
TBM	:	Tuberculous Meningitis
TD	:	Delay Time

TE	:	Time Echo
TI	:	Inversion Time
TIA	:	Transient Ischemic Attack
TMJ	:	Temporomandibular Joint
TOF	:	Time of Flight
TOPO	:	Topogram, Scanogram, Scout View, Pilot, Localizer
TPA	:	Tissue Plasminogen Activator
TR	:	Repetition Time
TS	:	Time Sequence
TW	:	Trigger Window
VB	:	Variable Bandwidth
VENC	:	Velocity Encoding
VR	:	Volume Rendering
W/L	:	Window Level
W/W	:	Window Width
WI	:	Weighted
XYZ	:	The Coordinate Axes of the rotating coordinate system

Index

S

T

U

V